Social Indicators Research Series

Volume 80

This series aims to provide a public forum for single treatises and collections of papers on social indicators research that are too long to be published in our journal *Social Indicators Research*. Like the journal, the book series deals with statistical assessments of the quality of life from a broad perspective. It welcomes research on a wide variety of substantive areas, including health, crime, housing, education, family life, leisure activities, transportation, mobility, economics, work, religion and environmental issues. These areas of research will focus on the impact of key issues such as health on the overall quality of life and vice versa. An international review board, consisting of Ruut Veenhoven, Ed Diener, Torbjorn Moum and Wolfgang Glatzer, will ensure the high quality of the series as a whole. Available at 25% discount for International Society for Quality-of-Life Studies (ISQOLS). For membership details please contact: ISQOLS; e-mail: office@isqols.org Editors: Ed Diener, University of Illinois, Champaign, USA; Wolfgang Glatzer, J.W. Goethe University, Frankfurt am Main, Germany; Torbjorn Moum, University of Oslo, Norway; Ruut Veenhoven, Erasmus University, Rotterdam, The Netherlands.

More information about this series at http://www.springer.com/series/6548

M. Joseph Sirgy

Positive Balance

A Theory of Well-Being and Positive Mental Health

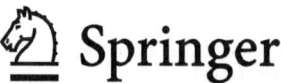 Springer

M. Joseph Sirgy
Virginia Polytechnic Institute and State University
Blacksburg, VA, USA

ISSN 1387-6570   ISSN 2215-0099   (electronic)
Social Indicators Research Series
ISBN 978-3-030-40288-4   ISBN 978-3-030-40289-1   (eBook)
https://doi.org/10.1007/978-3-030-40289-1

This Springer imprint is published by the registered company Springer Nature Switzerland AG.
The registered company address is: Gewerbestrasse 11, 6330 Cham, Switzerland

*This book is dedicated to my wife (Pamela),
my four children (Melissa, Danielle, Michelle,
and Emmaline), my four grandchildren
(Isabella, Alexander, Scott, and Jake), my two
brothers (Abraham and Jimmy), and my
cousins and their families scattered in the
USA, Canada, Australia, France, Lebanon,
and Egypt. The book is also dedicated to all
those well-being researchers who have
devoted much of their professional careers to
the promulgation of the science of well-being,
happiness, and quality of life—those who
believe that there is more to life than simply
surviving or minimizing the stresses and
strains of daily life. Well-being, happiness,
and quality-of-life researchers shine a beacon
of light to the science that can elevate human
existence and make people flourish.*

Preface

Here is a little history to help the reader better understand my personal motivation in writing this book. I am a management psychologist (Ph.D. in social/industrial/organizational psychology) and an endowed professor of marketing at Virginia Polytechnic Institute and State University. I have been a professor of marketing for the last 40 years and have written much about quality-of-life issues related to psychology, sociology, economics, political science, marketing, management, business ethics, corporate social responsibility, and public policy, among others.

Much of my early research has employed the concept of life satisfaction as a pivotal concept in several quality-of-life (QOL) research streams capturing aspects of material well-being, consumer well-being, employee well-being, residential well-being, and community well-being. I viewed life satisfaction as the primary concept that reflects well-being, and I treated it as the ultimate dependent variable. This perspective was clearly captured in my 2002 book on the *Psychology of Quality of Life* (Sirgy, 2002). In 2012, I published my second book on the *Psychology of Quality of Life* (Sirgy, 2012). The subtitle of that book was *Hedonic Well-Being, Life Satisfaction, and Eudaimonia*. At that time, I was able to document three major sets of well-being concepts, namely the three well-being concepts as captured in the book's subtitle. More recently, my colleagues and I have broadened our conceptualization of well-being to include these three concepts of well-being as articulated in the 2012 book, namely hedonic well-being (i.e., positive and negative affect), life satisfaction (overall life satisfaction as well as domain satisfaction), and eudaimonic well-being (i.e., personal growth, meaning in life, environmental mastery, self-actualization, social actualization, social integration, and social contribution)—addressed as dependent variables in various studies (Joshanloo, Sirgy, & Park, 2018a, 2018b).

In parallel, one of the research programs I carried out over the years dealt directly with the balanced life. My initial ideas of the balanced life were documented in my 2002 book on the psychology of quality of life (Sirgy, 2002; also see Sirgy, 2012). In that book, I wrote about how people achieve a balanced life by engaging in cognitive, affective, and behavior-based strategies dealing with satisfaction segmented in various life domains such as work life, family life, social life, and financial life. Specifically, I introduced two major balance principles: the principle of balance within life domains and the principle of balance between life domains. Balance within a life domain is achieved by experiencing both positive and negative events. Positive events serve a reward function. That is, goals are attained, and resources are acquired. Negative events serve a motivational function (i.e., these events lead the person to recognize problems and opportunities for further achievement and growth). In contrast, balance between life domains is achieved through compensation. Compensation takes two forms. One form involves the increase of the perceived importance or salience of life domains containing much positive affect to act as a countervailing force to life domains containing much negative affect. The second form involves the increase of salience of negative life domains to compensate for positive life domains. Increasing the importance of negative life domains motivates the individual to pay greater attention to that domain by prompting the individual to engage in corrective action within these domains. The goal is to decrease the negative valence of beliefs related to one's evaluation of the totality of a negative life domain.

I wrote (with one of my doctoral students) a paper (Sirgy & Wu, 2009) on that topic published in the *Journal of Happiness Studies*. This paper won the Best Paper Award in that journal and was reproduced in a book on happiness, edited by Antonella Delle Fave (Sirgy, 2013). In that paper, we argued that a balanced life (in addition to a pleasant life, an engaged life, and a meaningful life) contributes significantly to subjective well-being. Balance contributes to subjective well-being because of the satisfaction *limit* that people can derive from a single life domain. People must be involved in multiple domains to satisfy the full spectrum of human development needs. Different life domains tend to focus on different human developmental needs. More specifically, balance contributes to subjective well-being because subjective well-being can only be attained when both survival and growth needs are met. High levels of subjective well-being cannot be attained with satisfaction of basic needs or growth needs alone. Both sets of needs must be met to contribute significantly to subjective well-being.

In 2016, my colleague Dong-Jin Lee and I wrote a conceptual paper dealing with work-life balance (Sirgy & Lee, 2016). In that paper we identified four research streams that have well-articulated four corresponding factors in work-life balance: (1) balanced role commitment, (2) positive spillover, (3) role conflict, and (4) social alienation. Based on these four factors, we classified individuals into four work-life balance groups with differing levels of life satisfaction. We then explained the psychological dynamics of the model by articulating three balance principles: satisfaction spillover across life domains, need satisfaction quota, and satisfaction from basic plus growth needs.

In 2018, the same colleague (Dong-Jin Lee) and I reviewed much of the literature on work-life balance and developed an integrated model involving two key dimensions: engagement in work life and nonwork life and minimal conflict between social roles in work and nonwork life (Sirgy & Lee, 2018a). We cited much evidence suggesting that work-life balance has substantive consequences in terms of work-related, nonwork-related, and stress-related outcomes. We also identified a set of personal and organizational antecedents to work-life balance and explained their effects. Then, we described a set of theoretical principles to explain the effect of work-life balance on life satisfaction. These principles include satisfaction limits, satisfaction of the full spectrum of human developmental needs, role conflict, positive spillover, role enrichment, segmentation, and compensation. Doing so provided us with a solid foundation to further develop these theoretical principles of work-life balance, which were further articulated in another conceptual paper (Lee & Sirgy, 2018). In that paper, we proposed a formative conceptualization of work-life balance composed of a set of inter-life domain strategies used to increase life satisfaction. Specifically, work-life balance was conceptualized as a higher-order construct composed of four behavior-based life domain strategies and four cognition-based life domain strategies. The behavior-based strategies involve role engagement in multiple domains, role enrichment, domain compensation, and role conflict management. The cognition-based strategies involve positive spillover, segmentation, value compensation, and whole-life perspective. Our ideas of work-life balance were cultivated further to make the case of the balanced life in general in another book chapter in *e-Handbook of Subjective Well-Being* (Sirgy & Lee, 2018). We formally defined life balance as a state of equally moderate-to-high levels of satisfaction in important life domains contributing to life satisfaction. We argued that life balance is commonly achieved through two sets of inter-domain strategies, namely strategies to prompt greater participation of satisfied domains to contribute to life satisfaction and strategies to increase domain satisfaction and decrease dissatisfaction. Inter-domain strategies designed to prompt greater participation of satisfied life domains to contribute to life satisfaction include:

- Engagement in social roles in multiple life domains (explained by the principle of satisfaction limits)
- Engagement in roles in health, safety, economic, social, work, leisure, and cultural domains (explained by the principle of satisfaction of the full spectrum of human development needs)
- Engagement in new social roles (explained by the principle of diminishing satisfaction)
  Inter-domain strategies designed to increase domain satisfaction and decrease domain dissatisfaction include:

- Integrating domains with high satisfaction (explained by the principle of positive spillover)
- Optimizing domain satisfaction by changing domain salience (explained by the value-based compensation principle)
- Compartmentalizing domains with low satisfaction (explained by the segmentation principle)
- Coping with domain dissatisfaction by engaging in roles in other domains likely to produce satisfaction (explained by the behavior-based compensation principle)
- Stress management (explained by the principle of role conflict)
- Using skills, experiences, and resources in one role for other roles (explained by the principle of role enrichment)

In parallel, my colleagues and I used the concept of the balanced life to develop and test models of business ethics (e.g., Lee et al., 2014), the digital workplace (Lee & Sirgy, 2019), and marketing and retailing (e.g., Ekici, Sirgy, Lee, Yu, & Bosnjak, 2018; Lee et al., 2014; Sirgy, Lee, & Yu, 2020).

This work culminated in providing me with a foundation for my theory on positive balance. The foundation for the theory of positive balance was published in a recent article in *Quality of Life Research* (Sirgy, 2019). In that paper, I developed a hierarchical model of the balanced life (and positive mental health). I called it "positive balance." Specifically, I argued that individuals with positive balance are characterized to experience:

- A preponderance of neurochemicals related to positive emotions (dopamine, serotonin, etc.) relative to neurochemicals related to negative emotions (cortisol), at a physiological level
- A preponderance of positive affect (happiness, joy, etc.) relative to negative affect (anger, sadness, etc.), at an emotional level
- A preponderance of domain satisfaction (satisfaction in salient and multiple life domains such as family life and work life) relative to dissatisfaction in other life domains, at a cognitive level
- A preponderance of positive evaluations about one's life using certain standards of comparison (satisfaction with one's life compared to one's past life, the life of family members, etc.) relative to negative evaluations about one's life using similar or other standards of comparison, at a meta-cognitive level
- A preponderance of positive psychological traits (self-acceptance, personal growth, etc.) relative to negative psychological traits (pessimism, hopelessness, etc.), at a development level
- A preponderance of perceived social resources (social acceptance, social actualization, etc.) relative to perceived social constraints (social exclusion, ostracism, etc.), at a social-ecological level

This book is a direct extension of the Sirgy (2019) article. I further build the positive balance model by further articulating the concept of positive balance at the different hierarchical levels and developing the theoretical links between the hierarchical levels. This is my goal in writing this book. I hope that I met my goal. The reader will be the ultimate judge.

Blacksburg, VA, USA   M. Joseph Sirgy

References

Ekici, A., Sirgy, M. J., Lee, D-J., & Yu, G. B., & Bosnjak, M. (2018). The effects of shopping well-being and shopping ill-being on consumer life satisfaction. *Applied Research in Quality of Life, 13*(2), 333–353.

Joshanloo, M., Sirgy, M. J., & Park, J. (2018a). The importance of national levels of eudaimonic well-being to life satisfaction in old age: A global study. *Quality of Life Research, 27*(12), 3303–3311.

Joshanloo, M., Sirgy, M. J., & Park, P. (2018b). Directionality of the relationship between social well-being and subjective well-being: Evidence from a 20-year longitudinal study. *Quality of Life Research, 27*(8), 2137–2145.

Lee, D-J., & Sirgy, M. J. (2018). What do people do to achieve work-life balance? A formative conceptualization to help develop a metric for large-scale quality-of-life surveys. *Social Indicators Research, 138*(2), 771–791.

Lee, D-J., & Sirgy, M. J. (2019). Work-life balance in the digital workplace: The impact of schedule flexibility and telecommuting on work-life balance and overall life satisfaction. In M. Coetzee (Ed.), *Thriving in digital workspaces: Emerging issues for research and practice* (pp. 355–384). Dordrecht: Springer.

Lee, D-J., Yu, G. B., Sirgy, M. J., Ekici, A., Gurel-Atay, E., & Bahn, K. D. (2014). Shopping well-being and ill-being: Toward an integrated model. In F. Musso & E. Druica (Eds.), *Handbook of research on retailer-consumer relationship development* (pp. 27–44). Hershey, PA: IGI Global Publishing.

Lee, D-J., Yu, G. B., Sirgy, M. J., Singhapakdi, A., & Lucianetti, L. (2018). The effects of explicit and implicit ethics institutionalization on employee life satisfaction and happiness: The mediating effects of employee experiences in work life and moderating effects of work-family conflict. *Journal of Business Ethics, 147*(4), 855–874.

Sirgy, M. J. (2002). *The psychology of quality of life.* Dordrecht: Springer.

Sirgy, M. J. (2012). *The psychology of quality of life: Hedonic well-being, life satisfaction, and eudaimonia* (2nd edn). Dordrecht: Springer.

Sirgy, M. J. (2013). The pleasant life, the engaged life, and the meaningful life: What about the balanced life? In A. Dell Fave (Ed.), *The exploration of happiness* (pp. 175–192). Dordrecht: Springer.

Sirgy, M. J. (2019). Positive balance: A hierarchical perspective of positive mental health. *Quality of Life Research, 28*(7), 1921–1930.

Sirgy, M. J., & Lee, D-J. (2016). Work-life balance: A quality-of-life model. *Applied Research in Quality of Life, 11*(4), 1059–1082.

Sirgy, M. J., & Lee, D-J. (2018a). The psychology of life balance. In E. Diener, S. Oishi, & Louis Tay (Eds.), *e-Handbook of well-being: Noba Scholar Handbook series – Subjective well-being.* Salt Lake City, UT: DEF Publishers.

Sirgy, M. J., & Lee, D-J. (2018b). Work-life balance: An integrative review. *Applied Research in Quality of Life, 13*(1), 229–254.

Sirgy, M. J., Lee, D-J., & Yu, G. B. (2020). Shopping-life balance: Toward a unifying framework. *Applied Research in Quality of Life, 15*(1), 17–34.

Sirgy, M. J., & Wu, J. (2009). The pleasant life, the engaged life, and the meaningful life: What about the balanced life? *Journal of Happiness Studies, 10*(2), 183–196.

Acknowledgments

I am grateful to all my colleagues and friends who interacted with me discussing this important topic. Among them are my coauthors professors Dong-Jin Lee, Mohsen Joshanloo, Grace B. Yu, Michael Bosnjak, Jiyun Wu, Minyoung Kim, Ahmet Ekici, Anusorn Singhapakdi, and Eda Gurel-Atay.

I am most grateful to Alex Michalos, the editor of Springer's Social Indicators Research Book Series, who read the Sirgy (2019) article that was published in *Quality of Life Research* and encouraged me to further elaborate on the theoretical links between the hierarchical levels by writing this book. Alex Michalos has been my role model and a major source of inspiration since I first met him back in the early 1990s. I am equally grateful to Shinjini Chatterjee, senior editor at Springer who had enough confidence in me to produce a good book likely to make a lasting impact in our field of study, namely quality-of-life research. I am also grateful to Krithika Shivakumar and her production team at Springer for their excellent work in transforming the manuscript into a fine book.

I am additionally grateful to my family for moral support and love—my wife, Pamela Jackson, and my four daughters: Melissa Racklin (her husband Anton Racklin and her three beautiful children: Isabella, Alec, and Jake), Danielle Gray (and her son Scott), Michelle Sirgy, and Emmaline Smith. My many thanks are also extended to my two brothers, Abraham and Jimmy, and their families, as well as his many cousins and their families scattered in many places around the world.

About the Book

In the first chapter (Chap. 1: The Theory of Positive Balance in Brief), I briefly describe the theory at large. The theory can be summarized as follows. Individuals with high levels of well-being and positive mental health are characterized to experience (1) a preponderance of neurochemicals related to positive emotions (dopamine, serotonin, etc.) relative to neurochemicals related to negative emotions (cortisol), at a physiological level; (2) a preponderance of positive affect (happiness, joy, etc.) relative to negative affect (anger, sadness, etc.), at an emotional level; (3) a preponderance of domain satisfaction (satisfaction in salient and multiple life domains such as family life, work life, etc.) relative to dissatisfaction in other life domains, at a cognitive level; (4) a preponderance of positive evaluations about one's life using certain standards of comparison (satisfaction with one's life compared to one's past life, the life of family members, etc.) relative to negative evaluations about one's life using similar or other standards of comparison, at a meta-cognitive level; (5) a preponderance of positive psychological traits (self-acceptance, personal growth, etc.) relative to negative psychological traits (pessimism, hopelessness, etc.), at a development level; and (6) a preponderance of perceived social resources (social acceptance, social actualization, etc.) relative to perceived social constraints (social exclusion, ostracism, etc.), at a social-ecological level. Furthermore, well-being at each hierarchical level influences its superordinate constructs through emergence.

Chapter 2 (Positive Balance at the Physiological Level: Positive and Negative Neurotransmitters) advances the following definition of positive mental health at the physiological level. Individuals with high levels of well-being (specifically hedonic well-being) experience a preponderance of neurochemicals related to rewards (dopamine, serotonin, and oxytocin) relative to negative neurochemicals related to stress (cortisol), at a physiological level. This definition of positive mental health at the physiological level is based on much of the research literature on the neurobiology of hedonic well-being and the stress response system.

Chapter 3 (Positive Balance at the Emotional Level: Hedonic Well-Being) discusses the concept of positive balance at the emotional level of analysis. I define positive mental health at the emotional level as follows: Individuals with high levels of well-being experience a preponderance of positive emotions (happiness, joy, elation, contentment, serenity, etc.) relative to negative emotions (anger, hate, disgust, fear, jealousy, envy, etc.). This definition of positive mental health at the emotional level is based on much of the research related to three programs of research in well-being, namely the measurement of positive and negative affect, the broaden-and-build theory of positive emotions, and flow theory. How does well-being at the physiological level (neurochemicals associated with the reward system and stress) influence the formation of well-being at the emotional level (hedonic well-being)? Positive neurochemicals (dopamine, serotonin, and oxytocin) at the physiological level mediated by a process of cognitive appraisal result in positive affect (happiness, joy, contentment, etc.) at the emotional level; and conversely, negative neurochemicals (cortisol) mediated by a process of cognitive appraisal result in negative affect (anger, sadness, jealousy, envy, depression, etc.).

Chapter 4 (Positive Balance at the Cognitive Level: Domain Satisfaction) discusses the concept of positive balance at the cognitive level as reflected in domain satisfaction. I define positive mental health at the cognitive level as follows: Individuals characterized as having positive mental health tend to experience a preponderance of domain satisfaction (satisfaction in salient and multiple life domains such as family life, work life, and social life) relative to dissatisfaction in other life domains. This definition of positive mental health at the cognitive level is based on a program of research related to three balance principles: the principle of satisfaction limits, the principle of the full spectrum of human developmental needs, and the principle of diminishing satisfaction. How does well-being at the emotional level (hedonic well-being) influence the formation of well-being at the cognitive level (domain satisfaction)? I argue that positive and negative affect (at the emotional level) is mediated by a domain segmentation process to produce domain satisfaction.

Chapter 5 (Positive Balance at the Meta-Cognitive Level: Life Satisfaction) provides a definition of positive mental health based on the concept of positive balance at the meta-cognitive level. Individuals characterized as having positive mental health tend to experience a preponderance of positive evaluations about one's life using certain standards of comparison (satisfaction with one's life compared to one's past life, the life of family members, etc.) relative to negative evaluations about one's life using similar or other standards of comparison. I then discuss five programs of research supporting this definition of positive balance at the meta-cognitive level: multiple discrepancies theory, congruity life satisfaction, temporal life satisfaction, social comparison, frequency of positive affect, and homeostatically protected mood. I describe how domain satisfaction contributes to life satisfaction through an emergence process involving a bottom-up process. Specifically, domain satisfaction at the cognitive level, mediated by a bottom-up process at the meta-cognitive level, results in life satisfaction; and conversely, domain dissatisfaction mediated by a bottom-up process results in life dissatisfaction.

Chapter 6 (Positive Balance at the Developmental Level: Eudaimonia) offers a definition of positive mental health based on the concept of positive balance at the developmental level and discusses nine programs of research, supporting this definition: hedonic versus eudaimonic happiness, virtue ethics and balance, self-determination theory, personal expressiveness, psychological well-being, purpose and meaning in life, authentic happiness and orientations to happiness, flourishing, and resilience and satisfaction of the full spectrum of human needs. The definition is as follows: Individuals characterized as having positive mental health tend to experience a preponderance of positive psychological traits (self-acceptance, personal growth, purpose in life, environmental mastery, autonomy, positive relations with others, etc.) relative to negative psychological traits (pessimism, hopelessness, depressive disorder, neuroticism, impulsiveness, etc.). Following this discussion, I describe how positive balance expressed in eudaimonia (at the developmental level) is produced in part by life satisfaction (at the meta-cognitive level) mediated by a process involving personal growth and intrinsic motivation. Life satisfaction at the meta-cognitive level, mediated by a process involving high personal growth, results in high levels of eudaimonia at the developmental level; and conversely, life dissatisfaction mediated by a process involving low personal growth results in low levels of eudaimonia.

Chapter 7 (Positive Balance at the Social-Ecological Level: Socio-Eudaimonia) provides a definition of positive mental health based on the concept of positive balance at the social-ecological level: Individuals characterized as having positive mental health tend to experience a preponderance of social resources (social acceptance, social actualization, social contribution, social integration, social harmony, social belongingness, social attachment, familial attachment, etc.) relative to social constraints (social alienation, social discord, social exclusion, ostracism, etc.). Five programs of research support this definition of positive balance at social-ecological level: social well-being, social harmony, social belongingness, attachment theory, and social ostracism. I then describe how eudaimonia (at the developmental level) serves as a building block for socio-eudaimonia (at the social-ecological level). The key process involves a process involved in social and moral development. As such, I argue that high levels of eudaimonia at the developmental level, mediated by a process involving high social and moral development, result in high levels of socio-eudaimonia at the social-ecological level; and conversely, low levels of eudaimonia, mediated by a process involving low social and moral development, result in low levels of socio-eudaimonia.

In Chap. 8 (Concluding Thoughts) I provide the reader a brief synopsis of the theory. I discuss the emerging trend in positive psychology, coined as the "second wave." I then discuss two well-accepted definitions of quality of life, health, and mental well-being, namely the definitions provided by the WHO (1997) and Garlderisi et al. (2015). In doing so I compare these definitions to the definitions introduced in this book. Lastly, I compare selected models of mental health that involve hierarchical concepts of quality of life to my proposed theory: models proposed by Wilson and Cleary (1995), Dambrun et al. (2012), Huta and Waterman (2014), and Lomas, Hefferon, and Ivtzan (2015).

Contents

1 The Theory of Positive Balance in Brief..................... 1
  Introduction... 1
  Positive Mental Health as Positive Balance................... 7
    Positive Mental Health at the Physiological Level
    (Positive and Negative Neurotransmitters)................... 7
    Positive Mental Health at an Emotional Level (Hedonic Well-Being)... 11
    Positive Mental Health at the Cognitive Level (Domain Satisfaction)... 12
    Positive Mental Health at the Meta-Cognitive Level
    (Life Satisfaction)....................................... 14
    Positive Mental Health at the Developmental Level (Eudaimonia)... 16
    Positive Mental Health at the Social-Ecological Level (Socio-
    Eudaimonia)... 17
  Conclusion... 19
  References... 20

**2 Positive Balance at the Physiological Level: Positive and Negative
  Neurotransmitters**... 25
  Introduction... 25
  Programs of Research Supporting the Positive Balance Definition..... 27
    The Neurobiology of Hedonic Well-Being.................... 27
    The Stress Response System and Cortisol.................... 35
  Conclusion... 37
  References... 38

3 Positive Balance at the Emotional Level: Hedonic Well-Being...... 41
  Introduction... 41
  Programs of Research Supporting the Definition of Positive Balance... 43
    Positive and Negative Affect............................. 43
    Broaden-and-Build Theory of Positive Emotions............. 46
    Flow... 47
  Emergence... 48

Conclusion.   50
References.   51

4   Positive Balance at the Cognitive Level: Domain Satisfaction.   53
Introduction.   53
Life Balance.   55
Engagement in Social Roles in Multiple Life Domains
and the Principle of Satisfaction Limits.   58
Engagement in Roles in Health, Love, Family, Material, Social,
Work, Leisure, and Culture Domains; and the Principle
of Satisfaction of the Full Spectrum of Human
Developmental Needs.   60
Engagement in New Social Roles and the Principle of Diminishing
Satisfaction.   63
Emergence.   64
Conclusion.   68
References.   68

5   Positive Balance at the Meta-cognitive Level: Life Satisfaction.   73
Introduction.   73
Programs of Research Supporting the Positive Balance Definition.   74
Multiple Discrepancies.   74
Congruity Life Satisfaction.   78
Temporal Satisfaction.   80
Social Comparison.   82
Frequency of Positive Affect.   83
Homeostatically Protected Mood.   84
Emergence.   86
Conclusion.   89
References.   90

6   Positive Balance at the Developmental Level: Eudaimonia.   95
Introduction.   95
Programs of Research Supporting the Definition of Positive Balance. . .   98
Hedonic Versus Eudaimonic Happiness.   98
Virtue Ethics and Character Strengths. 100
Self-Determination Theory. 102
Personal Expressiveness. 104
Psychological Well-Being. 105
Purpose and Meaning in Life. 108
Authentic Happiness and Orientations to Happiness. 110
Flourishing. 112
Resilience. 113
Satisfaction of the Full Spectrum of Human Needs. 114
Emergence. 116
Conclusion. 118
References. 118

7 Positive Balance at the Social-Ecological Level: Socio-Eudaimonia 125
  Introduction 125
  Programs of Research Supporting the Positive Balance Definition 127
    Social Well-being 127
    Social Harmony 131
    The Need to Belong 133
    Attachment Theory 135
    Social Exclusion and Ostracism 136
  Emergence 137
  Conclusion 141
  References 142

8 Concluding Thoughts 145
  Introduction 145
  A Synopsis of the Theory 145
  Second Wave Positive Psychology 150
  Definitions of Quality of Life, Health, and Mental Well-being 151
  A Comparison of Models Involving Hierarchical Concepts
  of Quality of Life 152
    The Wilson/Cleary Model 152
    The Dambrun Model 153
    The Huta/Waterman Model 154
    The Lomas/Hefferon/Ivtzan Model 154
  Conclusion 155
  References 155

About the Author

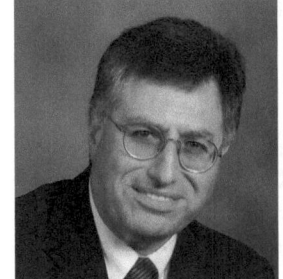

M. Joseph Sirgy is a management psychologist (Ph.D., U/Massachusetts, 1979) and the Virginia Tech Real Estate Professor of Marketing at Virginia Polytechnic Institute and State University (Virginia Tech). He has published extensively in the area of well-being and quality of life (QOL). He co-founded the International Society for Quality-of-Life Studies (ISQOLS) in 1995 and served as its Executive Director/Treasurer from 1995 to 2011 and as Development Co-Director (2011–2019). In 1998, he received the Distinguished Fellow Award from ISQOLS. In 2003, ISQOLS honored him as the Distinguished QOL Researcher for research excellence and a record of lifetime achievement in QOL research. He also served as President of the Academy of Marketing Science from which he received the Distinguished Fellow Award in the early 1990s and the Harold Berkman Service Award in 2007 (lifetime achievement award for serving the marketing professoriate). In the early 2000s, he helped co-found the Macromarketing Society and the Community Indicators Consortium and has served as a board member of these two professional associations. He co-founded the journal, *Applied Research in Quality of Life*, the official journal of the International Society for Quality-of-Life Studies, in 2005, and he served as co-founding editor (1995–present). He also served as editor of the QOL section in the *Journal of Macromarketing* (1995–2016). He received the Virginia Tech's Pamplin Teaching Excellence Award/Holtzman Outstanding Educator Award and University Certificate of Teaching Excellence in 2008. In 2010, ISQOLS honored him for excellence and lifetime service to the society. In 2010, he won the Best Paper Award in the *Journal of Happiness Studies* for his theory of the balanced life; in 2011, he won the Best Paper Award in the *Journal of Travel Research* for his goal theory of leisure travel satisfaction. In 2012, he was awarded the EuroMed Management Research Award for his outstanding achievements and groundbreaking contributions to well-being and quality-of-life research. In 2019, the Macromarketing Society honored him with the Robert W. Nason Award for extraordinary and sustained contributions to the field of macromarketing. He also was the editor of ISQOLS/ Springer book series on handbooks in QOL research, the community QOL indicators best practices, and applied quality-of-life research best practices and is currently the co-editor of human well-being and policy making and editor-in-chief of the *Journal of Macromarketing*. Among his recent books are:

- Sirgy, M. Joseph, Richard J. Estes, El-Sayed El-Aswad, and Don R. Rahtz (2019). *Combatting Jihadist Terrorism through Nation Building: A Quality-of-Life Perspective.* Dordrecht: Springer.
- Estes, Richard J. and M. Joseph Sirgy (2018). *Advances in Well-Being: Toward a Better World.* London: Rowman & Littlefield Publishers.
- Uysal, Muzaffer, Stefan Kruger, and M. Joseph Sirgy (Eds.) (2018). *Managing Quality of Life in Tourism and Hospitality: Best Practices.* Oxfordshire, UK: CABI Publishers.
- Estes, Richard J. and M. Joseph Sirgy (Eds.) (2017). *The Pursuit of Well-being: The Untold Global History.* Dordrecht, Netherlands: Springer Publishers.
- Sirgy, M. Joseph, Rhonda Phillips, and Don Rahtz (Eds.) (2013). *Community Quality-of-Life Indicators: Best Cases VI.* Dordrecht, Netherlands: Springer Publishers.
- Sirgy, M. Joseph (2012). *The Psychology of Quality of Life: Hedonic Well-Being, Life Satisfaction, and Eudaimonia.* 2nd edition. Dordrecht, Netherlands: Springer Publishers.

- Reilly, Nora P., M. Joseph Sirgy, and C. Allen Gorman (Eds.) (2012). *Work and Quality of Life: Ethical Practices in Organizations.* Dordrecht, Netherlands: Springer Publishers.
- Uysal, Muzaffer, Richard Perdue, and M. Joseph Sirgy (Eds.) (2012). *Handbook of Tourism and Quality-of-Life Research: Enhancing the Lives of Tourists and Residents.* Dordrecht, Netherlands: Springer Publishers.
- Land, Kenneth C., Alex C. Michalos, and M. Joseph Sirgy (Eds.) (2012). *Handbook of Social Indicators and Quality-of-Life Research.* Dordrecht, Netherlands: Springer Publishers.

List of Figures

Fig. 1.1   A hierarchical perspective of well-being   4

Fig. 2.1   Dopamine and serotonin pathways. Source: National Institutes
of Health, U.S. Department of Health and Human Services   28

Fig. 3.1   Emergence: well-being at the emotional level (positive/negative
affect) influenced by well-being at the physiological level (neurochemicals related to rewards and stress) mediated
by a process of cognitive appraisal   49

Fig. 4.1   Domain satisfaction strategies people use to create balance   58
Fig. 4.2   Emergence: well-being at the cognitive level (domain satisfaction)
influenced by well-being at the emotional level (hedonic
well-being) mediated by a process of domain segmentation   65

Fig. 5.1   Emergence: well-being at the meta-cognitive level (life satisfaction)
influenced by well-being at the cognitive level (domain satisfaction)
mediated by a process of bottom-up spillover   86
Fig. 5.2   How life satisfaction is determined through a bottom-up
process   88

Fig. 6.1   Emergence: Well-being at the developmental level (Eudaimonia)
influenced by well-being at the meta-cognitive level (life satisfaction) mediated by a process of personal growth
and intrinsic motivation   117

Fig. 7.1   Emergence: well-being at the social-ecological level (socio-
eudaimonia) influenced by well-being at the developmental level
(eudaimonia) mediated by a process of social and moral
development   141

List of Tables

Table 1.1   Positive mental health defined at various hierarchical levels
as positive balance with emergence 8

Table 2.1   Positive mental health defined at the physiological level 26

Table 3.1   Positive mental health defined at various hierarchical levels
as positive balance with emergence and focus
on the emotional level 42
Table 3.2   A scale measuring positive and negative affect 44
Table 3.3   Measuring hedonic sensations of momentary pleasures 45
Table 3.4   An emotional well-being scale 46

Table 4.1   Positive mental health defined at various hierarchical levels
as positive balance with emergence and focus on
the cognitive level 56
Table 4.2   Domains of life concerns 66

Table 5.1   Positive mental health defined at various hierarchical levels
as positive balance with emergence and focus
on the meta-cognitive level 75
Table 5.2   Ontological well-being 81
Table 5.3   The quality-of-life index 89

Table 6.1   Positive mental health defined at various hierarchical levels
as positive balance with emergence and focus
on the developmental level 97
Table 6.2   Ryff's psychological well-being measure 106
Table 6.3   Orientations to happiness 111
Table 6.4   The flourishing scale 113
Table 6.5   A need satisfaction hierarchy measure of well-being 115

Table 7.1   Positive mental health defined at various hierarchical levels
            as positive balance with emergence and focus
            on the social-ecological level   128

Table 8.1   Positive mental health defined at various hierarchical levels
            as positive balance with emergence   147

Chapter 1
The Theory of Positive Balance in Brief

Introduction

Mental health refers to the state of our emotional, psychological, and social well-being. It impacts the way we feel, think and act, making it important in all areas of our lives. Mental health plays an important role in the way we deal with stress, how we relate to others, and the decisions we make in our daily lives. Without positive mental health, it will be almost impossible to realize your full potential, work productively, make a meaningful contribution to your community, or handle the stress that comes with life. So, what can you do to ensure you have a healthy mental state? Well, there are various ways to maintain positive mental health and live a more fulfilling and enjoyable life. Besides seeking professional help if you need it, you should make time to connect with others, think positively about yourself and get physically active. Also, make sure you get enough rest, you're mindful of your present moment, and be helpful to others. A healthy mental state will help you leverage your Everyday Power to achieve the success you seek and live a purposeful life.—Norbert Juma (https://everydaypower.com/mental-health-quotes/)

My goal in this introductory chapter is to briefly flesh out the theory of positive balance. In the subsequent chapters, I will break down the discussion by each hierarchical level and provide much more detail concerning definitions of well-being at each level and the link between levels through a set of theoretical propositions capturing my understanding of much of the transdisciplinary research in well-being.

The literature of subjective well-being has blossomed considerably over the last five or six decades. Subjective well-being is traditionally defined as a broad category of phenomena that involves positive emotions (preponderance of positive over negative affect), domain satisfaction (satisfaction in various life domains such as family life, social life, work life, etc.), and life satisfaction (a global judgment of satisfaction with life overall) (see literature reviews in Allen, 2018; Dambrun et al., 2012; Diener, 1984; Diener, Suh, Lucas, & Smith, 1999; Kahneman, Diener, & Schwarz, 1999; Sirgy, 2012). Proponents of positive mental health (e.g., Keyes,

This chapter is adapted partly from Sirgy (2019).

© Springer Nature Switzerland AG 2020
M. J. Sirgy, *Positive Balance*, Social Indicators Research Series 80,
https://doi.org/10.1007/978-3-030-40289-1_1

2007) have long argued that much of the research in subjective well-being reflect a hedonic perspective of well-being. That is, the core concept reflects "feeling good about life" in various forms (preponderance of positive emotions, satisfaction with life domains, and satisfaction with life overall). However, the hedonic research tradition does not consider a parallel tradition of research involving eudaimonia. The eudaimonic tradition (e.g., Ryff, 1989) focuses on "functioning well in life." For example, eudaimonia (or psychological well-being) reflects the quality with which individuals are functioning in their lives (not necessarily and only how positive they feel about their lives). The construct involves at least five dimensions: (1) autonomy, (2) positive relations with others, (3) environmental mastery, (4) personal growth, and (5) purpose in life (cf. Ryan, Huta, & Deci, 2008; Ryff, 1989; Vitterso, 2016). Positive mental health researchers (e.g., Joshanloo, 2016; Joshanloo, Bobowick, & Basabe, 2016; Keyes, 1998, 2002, 2007, 2013; Keyes & Lopez, 2002; Keyes & Waterman, 2003; Robitschek & Keyes, 2009) have argued that positive mental health has to integrate the hedonic tradition with the eudaimonic tradition. They also explicitly introduced another major dimension of positive mental health, namely social well-being. Social well-being reflects positive social functioning. This construct involves at least five dimensions: (1) social acceptance, (2) social actualization, (3) social contribution, (4) social coherence, and (5) social integration. Hence, the focus of positive mental health in my theory of positive balance builds on the concept of positive mental health that incorporates aspects of subjective well-being, eudaimonia, and social well-being.

Before discussing the concept of positive mental health in detail, we first must make a clear distinction between mental well-being (or positive mental health) and mental ill-being (or psychopathology). This is important because the goal related to the study of positive mental health is essentially to enhance mental well-being or the quality of life of the individual, whereas the goal related to the study of mental ill-being focuses mostly on reducing psychopathology and mitigating dysfunction.[1] The focus here is on mental well-being, not mental-ill-being. Hence, I use the term mental well-being in this book in a manner consistent with Keyes' (1998, 2002, 2007, 2013) term of "positive mental health," to distinguish well-being aspects of mental health from the ill-being aspects (cf. Jahoda, 1958).

Much research has demonstrated this distinction clearly. For example, Headey, Holmstrom, and Wearing (1984) made the distinction between well-being and ill-being in their seminal article titled *Well-Being and Ill-Being: Different Dimensions*. The authors presented evidence that the construct of well-being is distinct from that of ill-being (i.e., the two constructs are not uni-dimensional). They were able to confirm this distinction using survey data involving four measures of well-being (Andrews and Withey's Life-as-a-Whole Index, the Self-Fulfillment Index, the

---

[1]In contrast, clinical psychology scholars have argued that the distinction between mental well-being and ill-being is counterproductive (e.g., Joseph & Wood, 2010). In essence, mental well-being should not be treated as a construct independent from mental ill-being. A continuum approach should be used in conceptualizing both mental well-being and ill-being, with positive functioning as one polar end of the continuum and negative functioning at the other end.

3-point Happy Scale, and Bradburn's Positive Affect Scale) and three measures of ill-being (Bradburn's Negative Affect Scale, the Worries Index, and the Somatic Complaints Index). Similarly, Lee and Oguzoglu (2004) used longitudinal survey data (the Household, Income, and Labour Dynamics in Australia Survey) to demonstrate the same point—that well-being and ill-being are not opposite ends of the same continuum. Their study found that while past ill-being had a significant impact on current well-being the reverse relationship is not true (i.e., past well-being did not have significant effect on current ill-being). To reiterate, the focus of my theory of positive balance is on mental "well-being," not mental "ill-being."

Although the accepted definition of positive mental health involving the dimensions of hedonic well-being, psychological well-being, and social well-being (e.g., Joshanloo, 2016; Joshanloo, Bobowick, & Basabe, 2016; Keyes, 1998, 2002, 2007, 2013; Keyes & Lopez, 2002; Keyes & Waterman, 2003; Robitschek & Keyes, 2009) is a good definition, it could be further refined to incorporate aspects of divergent set of concepts related to quality of life and well-being, such as:

- Stress response system (e.g., Lovallo, 2016; Sterling and Eyer 1988); neurobiology of well-being (e.g., Jackson, Sirgy, & Medley, 2018; Pressman & Cohen, 2005; Spinelli et al., 2012);
- Positive versus negative affect (e.g., Diener & Emmons, 1984; Diener et al., 2010); broaden and build theory (e.g., Fredrickson, 2001, 2004; Fredrickson & Joiner, 2002); and flow (e.g., Csikszentmihalyi & LeFevre, 1989);
- Principle of satisfaction limits (e.g., Lee & Sirgy, 2018; Sirgy & Lee, 2018a, 2018b; Sirgy & Wu, 2009); principle of the full spectrum of human developmental needs (e.g., Lee & Sirgy, 2018; Sirgy & Lee. 2018a, 2018b; Sirgy & Wu, 2009); principle of diminishing satisfaction (e.g., Lee & Sirgy, 2018; Sirgy & Lee, 2018a, 2018b; Sirgy & Wu, 2009);
- Multiple discrepancies theory (e.g., Michalos, 1985, 1986; Michalos et al., 2007); congruity life satisfaction (e.g., Meadow, Mentzer, Rahtz, & Sirgy, 1992; Sirgy et al., 1995); basis of life satisfaction judgments (e.g., Pavot & Diener, 1993; Suh, Diener, Oishi, & Triandis, 1998); social comparisons in life satisfaction (e.g., Frieswijk, Buunk, Steverink, & Slaets, 2004); frequency of life satisfaction judgments (e.g., Diener, Fujita, Tay, & Biswas-Diener, 2012);
- Virtue ethics and balance (e.g., Rowe & Broadie, 2002); self-determination theory (e.g., Ryan & Deci, 2000; Ryan, Huta, & Deci, 2008; Ryan & Martela, 2016), hedonic versus eudaimonic happiness (e.g., Deci & Ryan, 2008, Kahneman, Diener, & Schwarz, 1999), personal expressiveness (e.g., Huta & Waterman, 2014; Waterman, 1993), psychological well-being (e.g., Ryff, 1989); and
- Social well-being (e.g., Keyes, 1998, 2002, 2007, 2013), need to belong (e.g., Baumeister & Leary, 1995), attachment theory (e.g., Bretherton, 1985), social exclusion and ostracism (e.g., Wolfer & Scheithauer, 2013), and social harmony (e.g., Ho & Chan, 2009; Joshanloo & Weijers, 2014).

Based on the aforementioned concepts and related research, my theory of positive balance is designed to help integrate many of these disparate concepts of well-being by showing how various concepts of well-being are linked in a hierarchy of concepts

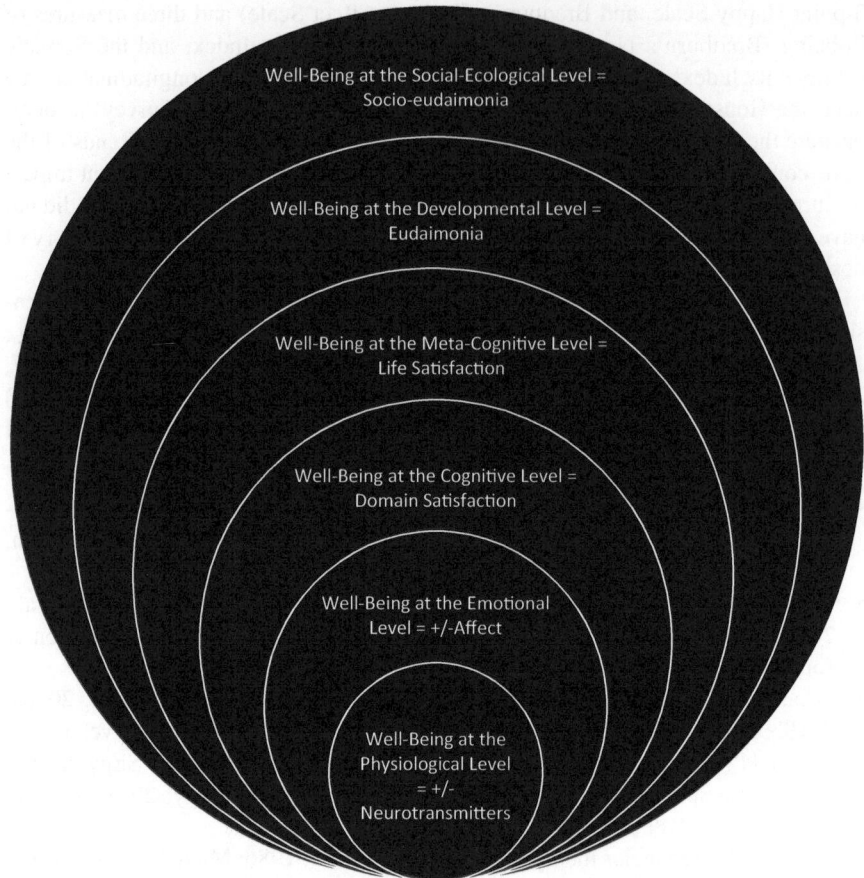

Fig. 1.1 A hierarchical perspective of well-being

capturing positive mental health. That is, well-being can best be construed in terms of a hierarchy of concepts varying from the most micro (physiological) to the most macro (social-ecological) (see Fig. 1.1). This hierarchical definition of positive mental health is guided by the concept of *positive balance* (a preponderance of a desirable state over an undesirable state specified at each level of analysis), which will be discussed briefly in this chapter and in some detail in subsequent chapters.

Before I begin describing positive mental health at each analytic level (i.e., physiological, emotional, cognitive, meta-cognitive, developmental, and social-ecological), I must articulate these different levels of analysis. The hierarchical concept of levels of analysis I use to describe various concepts of well-being is highly akin to the layering approach used by scholars of well-being (e.g., Dambrun et al., 2012; Huta & Waterman, 2014; Lomas, Hefferon, & Ivtzan, 2015). For example, Dambrun et al. (2012) used a hierarchical dimension varying from "fluctuating happiness" to "authentic-durable happiness." Fluctuating happiness is viewed as a micro-level concept that is ephemeral, temporary, and transient, whereas authentic-durable happiness is regarded as dispositional, stable, and enduring across a larger time frame. Similarly, Huta and Waterman (2014) distinguished among constructs of mental well-being based on a continuum in which the polar extremes are "state-like concepts" (most micro) to "trait-like concepts" (most macro). Furthermore, Lomas, Hefferon, and Ivtzan (2015) proposed a model of mental well-being using a similar layering scheme. Their LIFE model involved three dimensions (subjective/mind, objective/body, and social), each dimension containing five layers. The layers involved with the subjective/mind dimensions are embodiment (most micro) followed by emotions, cognition, consciousness, and awareness (most macro). The objective/body dimensions involve five hierarchy layers too: biochemistry (most micro), neurons, neural networks, nervous system, and the body at large (most macro). The social dimension also involve five hierarchical layers: microsystem (most micro), mesosystem, exosystem, macrosystem, and ecosystem (most macro).

To reiterate, my hierarchical layering involves six levels: (1) physiological, (2) emotional, (3) cognitive, (4) meta-cognitive, (5) developmental, and (6) social-ecological. The various levels of analysis reflect a continuum varying micro-level phenomena to macro ones. The most micro level analysis of well-being focuses on physiology. I begin by examining well-being based on the literatures involving biology, physiology, neurobiology, and medicine. At this level of analysis, I discuss well-being in terms of functional versus dysfunctional stress from a physiological perspective (i.e., concepts involving the autonomic and peripheral nervous system and the neurochemicals (e.g., dopamine, serotonin, norepinephrine, endorphins, oxytocin, cortisol, etc.) as they become excreted in response to stimuli from either the external or internal environments of the individual. Positive mental health at a physiological level is thus construed as a preponderance of neurochemical related to positive emotions (dopamine, serotonin, norepinephrine, endorphins, oxytocin, etc.) relative to neurochemicals related to negative emotions (cortisol, etc.). This is a physiological viewpoint of positive mental health because the focus is on the neurochemicals excreted as a function of daily events.

I call the second-level analysis "emotional" because it captures much of the well-being literature in terms of positive and negative affect. Positive mental health at the emotional level is thus construed as preponderance of positive affect (pleasure, happiness, joy, contentment, vitality, etc.) relative to negative affect (anger, sadness, jealousy, envy, hatred, grief, isolation, worthlessness, etc.). One can argue that the well-being concepts related to emotions (construed from the emotional-level perspective) are emergent from well-being concepts grounded in physiology. That is, positive and negative emotions are experienced when the individual engages in cognitive appraisal of these neurochemical surges. I discuss this concept of emergence in some detail in the following sections and in more detail throughout the book.

I then move to the cognitive level and describe well-being in terms of cognitive concepts involving life domains such as satisfaction with social life, family life, leisure life, financial life, work life, etc. One can argue that these cognitive judgments are emergent from positive and negative affect in relation to specific life domains resulting in domain satisfaction. The latter takes form in a cognitive evaluation based on affective experiences housed in the respective life domains. This is a cognitive process quality-of-life researchers commonly refer to as domain segmentation (i.e., segmenting emotional experiences in the form of life domains). As such, I view positive mental health at the cognitive level as a preponderance of satisfaction with salient and multiple life domains such as family life, work life, and leisure life, relative to dissatisfaction in other life domains.

Analysis of well-being at the meta-cognitive level involves a higher level of cognitions. Here, I discuss well-being in terms of life satisfaction, perceived quality of life, and other judgments of personal happiness. Again, one can argue that this level of analysis is one step elevated from domain satisfaction because cognitions related to life satisfaction are partly based on cognitions related to domain satisfaction. Hence, life satisfaction is emergent from domain satisfaction mediated by a process quality-of-life researchers commonly refer to as bottom-up spillover. At this level of analysis, I regard positive mental health as a preponderance of positive evaluations about one's life using certain standards of comparison (satisfaction with one's life compared to one's past life, the life of family members, the life of associates at work, the life of others in the same social circles, etc.) relative to negative evaluations about one's life using similar or other standards of comparison.

Moving up the hierarchy, I then focus on a developmental-level analysis of well-being, and at this level I describe concepts of well-being related to eudaimonia. These concepts are viewed as "developmental" because they are couched in a larger time frame, the life span—a time frame commonly used by most development psychologists. Again, one can argue that eudaimonia is an emergent concept from life satisfaction. That is, eudaimonia is predicated on life satisfaction mediated by a psychological process related to intrinsic motivation and personal growth. Thus, at a developmental level, positive mental health is treated as a preponderance of positive psychological traits (personal growth, purpose in life, environmental mastery, autonomy, positive relations with others, etc.) relative to negative psychological traits (pessimism, hopelessness, depressive disorder, neuroticism, impulsiveness, etc.).

Finally, I discuss well-being at the most macro level possible, the social-ecological level. In this context, well-being is described in terms of eudaimonia in a social context, a construct I refer to as "socio-eudaimonia." As such, positive mental health is construed at the social-ecological level as a preponderance of social resources (social acceptance, social actualization, social contribution, social integration, etc.) relative to social constraints (social exclusion, ostracism, etc.). Note that socio-eudaimonia is construed as an emergent phenomenon from eudaimonia (at the developmental level) mediated by a process of social and moral development (at the social-ecological level).

Positive Mental Health as Positive Balance

Given the preceding discussion I begin by offering an integrated definition of positive mental health. This definition is shown in Table 1.1 broken down by each level of analysis: physiological, emotional, cognitive, meta-cognitive, developmental, and social-ecological levels. Common across all levels of analysis is positive balance, *a preponderance of a desirable state over an undesirable state specified uniquely at each level of analysis.* Each definition of positive mental health, within its respective level of analysis, is discussed in the sections below.

Positive Mental Health at the Physiological Level (Positive and Negative Neurotransmitters)

Here is a positive balance definition of positive mental health at the physiological level: *Positive mental health is a state of mind in which is the individual experiences a preponderance of neurochemicals associated with the reward system (i.e., dopamine, serotonin, and oxytocin) relative to neurochemicals associated with stress (i.e., cortisol).*

Research in neuroscience has identified the major neurotransmitters implicated in positive affect: dopamine, serotonin, and oxytocin. In contrast, cortisol is associated with negative affect (see literature review by Jackson, Sirgy, & Medley, 2018). *Dopamine* plays a significant role in positive affect. It is the primary neurotransmitter operating in the brain reward system. All pleasurable activities (e.g., engaging in sexual intercourse, listening to music, eating and drinking when feeling hungry) are associated with the influx of dopamine. Reduced levels of *serotonin* are associated with negative mood, anxiety, and depression. *Oxytocin* is associated with maternal feelings as in childbirth and lactation, mother-infant bonding, and prosocial behavior.

Stress is customarily viewed as a state of physiological disharmony triggered by a stressor, psychological or physical threat. A psychological threat is usually a perceived adverse circumstance from the external environment (e.g., a physical attack by a predator) or it can originate internally as an infection or some other disease symptom (McEwen & Wingfield, 2003).

The endocrine response during stress involves two parallel responses: the adrenocortical response (involving the sympathetic nervous system) and the adrenomedullary response (involving the hypothalamus and pituitary) (Lovallo, 2016, pp. 57–62). The endocrine response during stress is regulated by *cortisol.* As such, homeostasis involves the regulatory action of cortisol, which is fundamental to normal functioning, daily activities, and survival in general. In contrast, allostasis involves repeatedly elevated and greatly prolonged high levels of cortisol (i.e., chronic stress), ultimately and adversely affecting mental well-being. This occurs through amygdala sensitization and loss of hippocampal volume, both

Table 1.1 Positive mental health defined at various hierarchical levels as positive balance with emergence

Level of analysis	Positive balance as positive mental health	Programs of research	Emergence
Positive mental health defined at a physiological level = **positive and negative neurotransmitters**	Individuals experiencing a preponderance of neurochemicals related to positive emotions (dopamine, serotonin, oxytocin) relative to neurochemicals related to negative emotions (cortisol)	Stress response system); neurobiology of happiness)	
Positive mental health defined at an emotional level = **positive/negative affect or hedonic wellbeing (positive/negative neurotransmitters + cognitive appraisals)**	Individuals experiencing a preponderance of positive emotions (happiness, joy, serenity, contentment, etc.) relative to negative emotions (anger, sadness, jealousy, envy, depression, etc.)	Positive versus negative affect; broaden and build theory; flow	Positive neurochemicals (dopamine, serotonin, and oxytocin) at the physiological level mediated by a process of cognitive appraisal (positive frame) result into positive affect (happiness, joy, contentment, etc.) at the emotional level; and conversely, negative neurochemicals (cortisol) mediated by a process of cognitive appraisal (negative frame) result into negative affect (anger, sadness, jealousy, envy, depression, etc.)
Positive mental health defined at a cognitive level = **domain satisfaction (positive/negative affect + domain segmentation)**	Individuals experiencing a preponderance of domain satisfaction (satisfaction in salient and multiple life domains such as family life, work life, social life, etc.) relative to dissatisfaction in other life domains	Principle of satisfaction limits; principle of the full spectrum of human developmental needs; principle of diminishing satisfaction	Positive affect (happiness, joy, contentment, etc.) at the emotional level mediated by a process of domain segmentation result into domain satisfaction (satisfied with work life, social life, family life, etc.); and conversely, negative affect (anger, sadness, jealousy, envy, depression, etc.) mediated by a

(continued)

Table 1.1 (continued)

Level of analysis	Positive balance as positive mental health	Programs of research	Emergence
			process of domain segmentation result into domain dissatisfaction (dissatisfied with work life, social life, family life, etc.)
Positive mental health defined at a meta-cognitive level = **life satisfaction (domain satisfaction + bottom-up process)**	Individuals experiencing a preponderance of positive evaluations about one's life using certain standards of comparison (satisfaction with one's life compared to one's past life, the life of family members, the life of associates at work, the life of others in the same social circles, etc.) relative to negative evaluations about one's life using similar or other standards of comparison	Multiple discrepancies theory; congruity life satisfaction; temporal life satisfaction; social comparison; frequency of positive affect; homeostatically protected mood	Domain satisfaction (satisfied with work life, social life, family life, etc.) at the cognitive level mediated by a bottom-up process at the meta-cognitive level result in life satisfaction; and conversely. domain dissatisfaction (dissatisfied with work life, social life, family life, etc.) mediated by a bottom-up process result in life dissatisfaction
Positive mental health defined at a developmental level = **eudaimonia (life satisfaction + personal growth)**	Individuals experiencing a preponderance of positive psychological traits (self-acceptance, personal growth, purpose in life, environmental mastery, autonomy, positive relations with others, etc.) relative to negative psychological traits (pessimism, hopelessness, depressive disorder, neuroticism, impulsiveness, etc.)	Hedonic versus eudaimonic happiness; virtue ethics and character strengths; self-determination theory; personal expressiveness; psychological well-being; purpose and meaning in life; flourishing; orientations to happiness; resilience; and satisfaction of the full spectrum of human needs	Life satisfaction at the meta-cognitive level mediated by a process involving high personal growth result in high levels of eudaimonia at the developmental level; and conversely, life dissatisfaction mediated by a process involving low personal growth result into low levels of eudaimonia
Positive mental health defined at a social-ecological level = **socio-eudaimonia (eudaimonia + social & moral development)**	Individuals experiencing a preponderance of social resources (social acceptance, social actualization, social contribution, social integration, social harmony, social	Social well-being, social harmony need to belong, attachment theory; social exclusion and ostracism	High levels of eudaimonia at the developmental level mediated by a process involving high social and moral development result into high levels of

(continued)

Table 1.1 (continued)

Level of analysis	Positive balance as positive mental health	Programs of research	Emergence
	belongingness, social attachment, familial attachment, etc.) relative to social constraints (social alienation, social discord, social exclusion, ostracism, etc.)		socio-eudaimonia at the social-ecological level; and conversely, low levels of eudaimonia mediated by a process involving low social and moral development result into low levels of socio-eudaimonia

associated with the formation and consolidation of long-term memory of adverse events (Lovallo, 2016, p. 132). Specifically, when the amygdala is exposed to chronic stress it becomes sensitized to aversive or threatening stimuli rendering the entire central nervous system highly reactive to fight-or-flight events. This *amygdala-sensitization effect* is associated with post-traumatic stress disorder (e.g., Bremner et al., 1995). In other words, stress-induced changes in cognition and memory exert a long-term effect on stress reactivity and well-being (both physiological and psychological). Repeatedly elevated and greatly prolonged high levels of cortisol is also associated with *shrinkage of hippocampal volume* (e.g., Gilbertson et al., 2002). Patients with post-traumatic stress disorder have reduced hippocampal volume. The hippocampus is the primary site of negative feedback for cortisol regulation. Also, it is important to note that disease, frailty, and disability have a direct toll of the stress response in that individuals afflicted with disease, frailty, and/or disability are likely to experience allostasis—continuing force acting against homeostasis causing the individual to continually expend additional resources to maintain homeostasis but at a systemic cost on mental well-being (e.g., McEwen & Wingfield, 2003; Rockwood, Hogan, & MacKnight, 2000).

Much research has demonstrated that positive emotions serve as stress buffers the deleterious effects of stress on the immune system (see literature review in Hostinar & Gunnar, 2013). For example, social stress, especially early in life, produces high levels of cortisol responses during social interactions and long-standing reductions in serotonin levels, underscoring the relationship between neurochemicals associated with positive and negative emotions (Spinelli et al., 2012). In a meta-analytic study, Pressman and Cohen (2005) found a negative relationship between dispositional positive affect and cortisol—the higher the dispositional positive affect the lower the cortisol.

Positive Mental Health at an Emotional Level (Hedonic Well-Being)

Well-being scientists (e.g., Diener & Emmons, 1984) tend to view subjective well-being partly as a psychological state involving a preponderance of positive affect (e.g., joy, contentment, pleasure) over negative affect (e.g., sadness, depression, anxiety, anger). The *broaden-and-build theory of positive emotions* (e.g., Fredrickson, 2001, 2004; Fredrickson & Joiner, 2002) asserts that positive emotions broaden an individual's momentary thought-action repertoire. Positive emotions induce playfulness, exploratory behavior, savoring experiences, creativity, close connections and bonding with others, among other positive behavioral outcomes. In contrast, negative emotions (associated with the visceral fight-or-flight response) prompt the individual to contract behaviorally. The broadening of the thought-action repertoire through positive emotions allows the individual to build personal resources—physical resources, intellectual resources, social resources, psychological resources, etc. These resources serve the individual in many ways to enhance functioning. Furthermore, these resources serve as reserves that can be drawn on to help deal with adverse events. As such, these resources enhance resilience. There is evidence to suggest that it is not only positive emotions that produce positive behavioral outcomes but the preponderance of positive affect over negative affect (Fredrickson, 2009, 2013). People who "flourish" (those who are psychologically healthy and satisfied with life) experience at least three times as many positive emotions as they do negative emotions. In contrast, the ratio is two-to-one for "nonflourishers."

But then the question is whether positive emotions contribute to positive mental health in a linear fashion. Research has addressed this question, and the answer is a resounding no. Too much positivity is not necessarily good for positive mental health. See discussion of this research question and evidence in Forgas (2014) and Fredrickson and Joiner (2002). The relationship looks more like an inverted-U. Too much positive emotions do not contribute to high levels mental well-being. Fredrickson (2013) argues that increasing positivity contributes to creativity, job performance, health, and other outcomes up to a certain level. After moderate levels of positive emotions, these behavioral outcomes diminish significantly. It has been demonstrated that some degree of negative emotions is necessary to motivate people to take corrective action. Corrective action leads to positive behavioral outcomes (Catalino, Algoe, & Fredrickson, 2011; Fredrickson, 2013). This evidence points to the assertion that positive mental health reflects a preponderance of positive over negative emotions. That is, negative emotions must be part of this optimal state but significantly in lesser amount than positive emotions.

Besides the research on the broaden-and-build theory, much of the research on *flow* reflects the notion that well-being is associated with both positive and negative emotions (e.g., Csikszentmihalyi & LeFevre, 1989). Specifically, certain activities that are challenging and matching one's level of skills induce much positive emotions (positive emotions related to achievement, mastery, and efficacy) juxtaposed with negative emotions (frustration related to task difficulty, pain in the exertion of physical and mental effort, and perseverance in light of failure). Engaging in activities that produce flow contributes significantly to life satisfaction. Note that flow theory emphasizes the notion that the flow experience necessitates elements that call for negative affect (i.e., physical exertion, effort, and learning from failure experiences). As such, here is a positive balance definition of positive mental health at the emotional level. *Positive mental health is a state of mind in which the individual experiences a preponderance of positive emotions (pleasure, happiness, joy, contentment, vitality, etc.) relative to negative emotions (anger, sadness, jealousy, envy, hatred, grief, isolation, worthlessness, etc.).*

How does well-being at the physiological level (positive and negative neuro-chemicals) contribute to the formation and maintenance of well-being at the emotional level (positive and negative affect)? This occurs through emergence. Emergence is a concept well-entrenched in systems science, especially in biology and the life sciences (Aderem, 2005; Crommelinck, Feltz, & Goujon, 2006; Solé, Ferrer-Cancho, Montoya, & Valverde, 2002). Specifically, emergence refers to higher-level systems "emerge" from lower-level systems. In other words, complex systems have "emergent properties" that are not inherent in their individual parts and cannot be understood even with full understanding of the parts alone. For example, understanding the properties of hydrogen and oxygen does not allow us to understand the properties of water. Also, life as we know it is an example of an emergent property. It is not inherent in DNA, cells, or organs but is a consequence of their actions and interactions.

As such, positive and negative affect (or hedonic well-being), commonly treated as the key concept of well-being at the emotional level, is an emergent property of positive and negative neurochemicals in the brain mediated by a process of cognitive appraisal. Much research has demonstrated that emotions are the direct result of cognitive appraisal of surges of neurochemicals in the brain (e.g., Denson, Spanovic, & Miller, 2009). That is, the cognitive appraisal of surges of positive neurotransmitters in the brain (dopamine, serotonin, and oxytocin) at the physiological level result in the experience of positive affect (joy, elation, contentment, happiness, serenity, etc.) at the emotional level. Conversely, cognitive appraisal of surges of negative neurotransmitters (cortisol) at the physiological level result in the experience of negative affect (anger, sadness, jealousy, envy, depression, etc.) at the emotional level.

Positive Mental Health at the Cognitive Level (Domain Satisfaction)

Early quality-of-life researchers (e.g., Andrews & Withey, 1976; Campbell, Converse, & Rodgers, 1976) have long acknowledged that affect is segmented in life domains such as family life, social life, work life, leisure life, community life, etc.

This is referred to as "domain satisfaction." That is, individuals can judge the level of satisfaction they have with various life domains—satisfaction with family life, social life, work life, leisure life, etc. Individuals make judgments about their life satisfaction overall based on domain satisfaction (see review of this literature in Sirgy, 2012).

I believe that positive mental health is achieved through positive balance in multiple domain satisfaction—that is, the individual experiences moderate-to-high satisfaction not only in one domain but with a range of domains. Positive mental health cannot be achieved from satisfaction in a single domain. Satisfaction must derive from multiple domains. This assertion is supported by much theory and research (see Lee & Sirgy, 2018; Sirgy & Lee, 2016, 2018a, 2018b; Sirgy & Wu, 2009 for extended discussions) and is articulated through three major principles: the principle of satisfaction limits, the principle of satisfaction of the full spectrum of human development needs, and the principle of diminishing satisfaction.

Specifically, the *principle of satisfaction limits* (e.g., Lee & Sirgy, 2018; Sirgy & Lee, 2016, 2018a, 2018b; Sirgy & Wu, 2009) asserts that the amount of contribution of domain satisfaction from a single life domain to life satisfaction is limited. That is, high role engagement in a single life domain with little or no role engagement in other life domains cannot contribute much to life satisfaction, compared to high role engagement in multiple domains. Individuals who have a high level of role engagement in life domains related to both basic needs (e.g., health, love, family, and material domains) and growth needs (e.g., social, work, leisure, and culture domains) are likely to experience greater satisfaction among life domains contributing to higher life satisfaction than those who have a high level of role engagement in domains related to only basic or growth needs. This effect is explained through the *principle of satisfaction of the full spectrum of human developmental needs* (e.g., Lee & Sirgy, 2018; Sirgy & Lee, 2016, 2018a, 2018b; Sirgy & Wu, 2009). The combined and balanced effects of satisfaction of both basic and growth needs serve to contribute to life satisfaction. That is, satisfaction of the full spectrum of human developmental needs (balance between basic and growth need satisfaction) produces the highest level of life satisfaction.

The *principle of diminishing satisfaction* (e.g., Lee & Sirgy, 2018; Sirgy & Lee, 2016, 2018a, 2018b; Sirgy & Wu, 2009) posits that people become engaged in new social roles to mitigate decreases in domain satisfaction and life satisfaction overall. This effect is due to diminishing satisfaction associated with a social role. That is, those who are engaged in social roles experience diminishing satisfaction in each life domain over time, which in turn detract from life satisfaction. To guard against this diminishing domain satisfaction, people engage in new social roles to generate new satisfaction, thereby compensating for the diminished satisfaction related to the old roles.

The preceding discussion points to the notion that positive mental health is associated with satisfaction in multiple life domains such as family life, work life, and leisure life. To enhance mental well-being, individuals invest much effort and energy in salient and multiple life domains to generate much needed positive affect to meet their human developmental needs, both basic and growth needs. As such, a reasonable definition of positive mental health at the cognitive level can be stated as follows: *Positive mental health is a state of mind in which the individual experiences a preponderance of domain satisfaction (satisfaction in salient and multiple life domains such as family life, work life, social life, etc.) relative to dissatisfaction in other life domains.*

How does well-being at the emotional level (i.e., positive/negative affect or hedonic well-being) contribute to the formation and maintenance of well-being at the cognitive level (domain satisfaction)? Again, this occurs through emergence. As explained in the previous section, emergence refers to higher-level systems "emerging" from lower-level systems. For example, understanding the properties of hydrogen and oxygen does not allow us to understand the properties of water. As such, domain satisfaction, commonly treated as the key concept of well-being at the cognitive level, is an emergent property of positive and negative affect mediated by a cognitive process of domain segmentation. Much research has demonstrated that people make evaluations of their various life domains (e.g., Andrews & Withey, 1976; Campbell, Converse, & Rodgers, 1976). Survey respondents are commonly asked to express how they feel about their work life, family life, social life, etc. These evaluations of their life domains are referred to as *domain satisfaction*. That is, positive affect (happiness, joy, contentment, etc.) at the emotional level mediated by a process of domain segmentation result into domain satisfaction (satisfied with work life, social life, family life, etc.); and conversely, negative affect (anger, sadness, jealousy, envy, depression, etc.) mediated by a process of domain segmentation result into domain dissatisfaction (dissatisfied with work life, social life, family life, etc.)

Positive Mental Health at the Meta-Cognitive Level (Life Satisfaction)

Life satisfaction is a concept that has been well-documented in the literature of quality-of-life studies and well-being research; see an extensive description of this concept and related research in much of the research by Diener and his colleagues (see literature review Diener, 1984; Diener et al., 1999). Life satisfaction is one of the four dimensions of subjective well-being. The other three are domain satisfaction, preponderance of positive over negative affect, and the absence of feelings of ill-being. Life satisfaction involves a cognitive evaluation of one's own life. Many large-scale social surveys use the following item to capture life satisfaction: "How satisfied or dissatisfied are you with your life overall? Very dissatisfied (1), Somewhat dissatisfied (2), So/so (3), Somewhat satisfied (4), and Very satisfied (5)." See examples of life satisfaction metrics in Sirgy (2012, Chapter 1 and Appendix).

Life satisfaction is essentially an evaluation that an individual makes about his or her life at large, and that this evaluation is a judgment which is strongly influenced by the type of cognitive frame used in decision-making (i.e., standard of comparisons or cognitive referents). That is, the individual judges his or her life against some standard (Day, 1987). This standard of comparison is selected and defined by the individual. It may involve a comparison of one's current life circumstance with old circumstances, a comparison of current life experience with prior expectations, etc.

A widely accepted theory related to how individuals make life satisfaction judgments is *multiple discrepancies theory* (Michalos, 1985, 1986; Michalos et al., 2007). The theory posits that overall life satisfaction is inversely proportional to the perceived differences between what one has versus seven different standards of comparisons. These are:

1. What one wants
2. What others have
3. The best one has had in the past
4. What one expected to have 3 years ago
5. What one expects to have in 5 years
6. What one deserves
7. What one needs

Congruity life satisfaction theory (Meadow et al., 1992; Sirgy et al., 1995) is akin to multiple discrepancies theory. The central tenet of this theory is that life satisfaction is function of comparison between perceived life accomplishments and a set of standards, namely standards related to derivative sources (accomplishments of relatives, friends, and associates; past accomplishments, average person in a similar occupation, etc.) and different forms (one's view of the ideal life, the deserved life, the minimum tolerable life, etc.).

Research on *temporal life satisfaction* (e.g., Pavot, Diener, & Suh, 1998) has also demonstrated that individuals make life satisfaction judgments based on their assessment of their own past, present, and future strivings. Other research has shown that the life satisfaction judgment is mostly determined by evaluations of one's life circumstances in relation to different standards of comparisons: one's belief in an ideal life such as one's aspirations of material acquisitions (e.g., Pavot & Diener, 1993), cultural norms such as being wealthy is a sign of happiness in life (e.g., Suh et al., 1998), social comparisons such as comparing one's life circumstances against the circumstances of one's siblings (e.g., Frieswijk et al., 2004), etc.

The point of this discussion is to underscore the notion that life satisfaction judgments are made using various standards of comparison. Positive mental health is influenced by the frequency and positivity of life satisfaction judgments–the more frequent and positive these judgments are the more positive the mental health of the individual (Diener et al., 2012). As such, I can offer a definition of positive mental health at the meta-cognitive level as follows: *Positive mental health is a state of mind in which the individual experiences a preponderance of positive evaluations about one's life using certain standards of comparison (satisfaction with one's life compared to one's past life, the life of family members, the life of associates at work, the life of others in the same social circles, etc.) relative to negative evaluations about one's life using similar or other standards of comparison.*

How does well-being at the cognitive level (domain satisfaction) contribute to the formation and maintenance of well-being at the meta-cognitive level (life satisfaction)? Again, this occurs through emergence. As explained in the two preceding sections, emergence refers to higher-level systems "emerging" from lower-level systems. As such, life satisfaction, commonly treated as the key concept of well-being at the meta-cognitive level, is an emergent property of domain satisfaction mediated by a bottom-up spillover process. Much research has demonstrated that people make life satisfaction judgments (e.g., Andrews & Withey, 1976; Campbell, Converse, & Rodgers, 1976). Survey respondents are commonly asked to express how they feel about their life in general. These evaluations of their life overall are referred to as *life satisfaction*. That is, domain satisfaction (satisfied with work life, social life, family life, etc.) at the cognitive level mediated by a bottom-up spillover process at the meta-cognitive level result in life satisfaction; and conversely, domain dissatisfaction (dissatisfied with work life, social life, family life, etc.) mediated by a bottom-up process result in life dissatisfaction.

Positive Mental Health at the Developmental Level (Eudaimonia)

The classic Greek philosopher, Aristotle, in *Nichomachean Ethics*, written in 350 B. C., provided guidance about how to live a good life, an ethical life (Rowe & Broadie, 2002). Happiness is not necessarily about pleasure. It is about virtue, and virtue is essentially life balance—balance applied to many areas of living. For example, balance in material life is balance between material excess and material deficiency. Too much honor leads to vanity and too little turns to undue humility. Too much amusement becomes buffoonery, too little is dullness. The principle of balance as virtue is to choose deliberate action that avoids both excess and deficiency. Virtue also involves activities that have significant life purpose.

Well-being researchers have distinguished between two major dimensions of well-being, namely hedonic and eudaimonic well-being (e.g., Deci & Ryan, 2008). The hedonic conception of well-being treats well-being in terms of life satisfaction, domain satisfaction, the preponderance of positive over negative affect, as well as the absence of feelings of depression (Diener, 1984; Diener et al., 1999). In contrast, the eudaimonic conception of well-being treats well-being in terms of personal growth and development—cognitive, emotional, social, and moral growth. As such, it is viewed as the cornerstone of positive mental health (e.g., Delle Fave, Brdar, Freire, Vella-Brodrick, & Wissing, 2011; Duckworth & Gross, 2014; Munoz Sastre, 1998; Ryan & Deci, 2000; Ryan, Huta, & Deci, 2008; Schwartz, 2015; Schwartz and Wrzesniewski 2016; Vitterso, 2016; Waterman, 1993). As such, eudaimonic well-being can be considered as a concept emergent from subjective well-being, and there is much evidence suggesting that the two concepts are correlated but nevertheless distinct (e.g., Joshanloo, 2016). Ryff's (1989) concept of psychological well-being captures a reasonable conceptualization of eudaimonia. Psychological well-being reflects personal growth and development. The construct of psychological well-being involves personal growth, purpose in life, environmental mastery, autonomy, and positive relations with others.

The preceding discussion emphasizes the need to consider psychological traits of the individual to better appreciate the concept of positive mental health. Positive psychological traits, such as personal growth and purpose in life, adds substantially to mental well-being. Conversely, negative psychological traits such as pessimism and neuroticism play a significant deleterious role in mental well-being. As such, my definition of positive mental health at the developmental level is as follows: *Positive mental health is characterized by individuals who have high levels of eudaimonia. This state of mind is mostly determined by a preponderance of positive psychological traits (personal growth, purpose in life, environmental mastery, autonomy, and positive relations with others, etc.) relative to negative psychological traits (pessimism, hopelessness, depressive disorder, neuroticism, impulsiveness, etc.).*

How does well-being at the meta-cognitive level (i.e., life satisfaction) contribute to the formation and maintenance of well-being at the developmental level (i.e., eudaimonia)? Again, this occurs through emergence. To remind the reader, emergence refers to higher-level systems "emerging" from lower-level systems. As such, eudaimonia, commonly treated as the key concept of well-being at the developmental level, is an emergent property of life satisfaction mediated by a process involving intrinsic motivation and personal growth (Deci & Ryan, 2008; Ryff, 1989). Much research has demonstrated that eudaimonia and life satisfaction are interrelated (e.g., Keyes, Shmotkin, & Ryff, 2002). Eudaimonia is not the same as life satisfaction. Eudaimonia builds on life satisfaction by bringing in other elements related to developmental psychology such as ego-development. In sum, life satisfaction at the meta-cognitive level mediated by a process involving intrinsic motivation and personal growth results in high levels of eudaimonia at the developmental level; and conversely, life dissatisfaction mediated by a process involving low personal growth results into low levels of eudaimonia.

Positive Mental Health at the Social-Ecological Level (Socio-Eudaimonia)

The most popular definition of positive mental health involves a multidimensional construct with three major constructs: hedonic well-being, psychological well-being, and social well-being (Keyes, 1998, 2002, 2007, 2013). Hedonic well-being involves positive affect, life satisfaction, as well as the absence of negative affect. This construal of hedonic well-being is essentially synonymous with subjective well-being (e.g., Diener, 1984; Diener et al., 1999). I discussed these as concepts of well-being at lower levels of analysis (emotional, cognitive, and meta-cognitive levels). As described in the preceding section, psychological well-being focuses on personal growth and development. It involves positive psychological traits such as personal growth, purpose in life, environmental mastery, autonomy, and positive relations with others. The construct of psychological well-being is essentially based on Ryff's (1989) model of psychological well-being. In contrast, *social well-being* reflects positive aspects of human well-being through interaction with other people and the community at large. This construct involves at least five dimensions (e.g., Keyes, 1998, 2002, 2003: Keyes & Lopez, 2002, Keyes & Waterman, 2003; Robitschek & Keyes, 2009): (1) social acceptance (i.e., a positive view of people and human nature), (2) social actualization (i.e. a positive view of human society and human strivings to elevate civil society), (3) social contribution (i.e., a positive view of the need to contribute to society through good deeds), (4) social coherence (i.e., a positive view of how institutions work to foster societal well-being), and (5) social integration (i.e., a positive view of social identity and a sense of belonging to a community). Research has demonstrated that subjective well-being, psychological well-being, and social well-being are correlated but also are empirically distinct (e.g., Gallagher, Lopez, & Preacher, 2009; Joshanloo 2016; Joshanloo, Bobowick, & Basabe, 2016; Keyes, 2002; Keyes, Shmotkin, & Ryff, 2002; Robitschek & Keyes, 2009; Shapiro & Keyes, 2008).

The concept of social well-being is consistent with a large literature in cross-cultural psychology on *social harmony* (e.g., Ho & Chan, 2009; Joshanloo & Weijers, 2014). Social harmony is important in the way the individual adapts to the environment. Social harmony can be described as social quality, which means social-economic security, social inclusion, social cohesion, and empowerment in developing the individual's potential. For example, people in collectivistic societies adapt better to their environment by engaging in behaviors considered "collective" such as teamwork and sharing credit for successful task completion and blame for task failure. Morling and Fiske (1999) viewed social harmony in terms of the individual recognizing that control resides in contextual and social forces. As such, the individual attempts to merge with these forces, accepting his or her role and the social norms that guide his or her performance in these roles. Carlquist, Ulleberg, Delle Fave, Nafstad, and Blakar (2017) were able to show that Norwegians' perceptions of happiness and the good life can be categorized in terms of two key dimensions: internal and external. The external dimension involves a variety of happiness concepts related to social relationships, whereas the internal dimension focuses on the individual own emotional experiences. The effect of age was a key finding. Young people view happiness in relation to an internal conception of happiness, whereas older people view happiness in terms of the external dimension. In other words, as people age, their conception of happiness turns from inward to outward. This finding reinforces the notion that a holistic view of positive mental health should include both self and social dimensions. Bauer (2016) also emphasized the distinction between "internalist" and "externalist" beneficiaries of the good life. The internalist beneficiary of the good mostly involves hedonic pleasures (i.e., positive and negative affect, life satisfaction, self-esteem, and hedonic motives) and eudaimonic meaning (i.e., psychological well-being, meaning in life, satisfaction of agentic needs, individual authenticity, and self-efficacy). In contrast, the externalist beneficiary of the good life involves eudaimonic meaning in the form of positive relations with others, social well-being, flourishing, satisfaction with communal needs, social authenticity, and identity status commitment.

Much of this discussion hints at a possible imperative: the need to consider the social resources available in one's environment as well as social constraints. As such, positive mental health at the social-ecological level of analysis can be defined as follows: *Positive mental health is a state of mind in which the individual experiences a preponderance of social resources (social acceptance, social actualization, social contribution, social coherence, social integration, etc.) relative to social constraints (social exclusion, ostracism, etc.).*

How does well-being at the development level (i.e., eudaimonia) contribute to the formation and maintenance of well-being at the social-ecological level (i.e., socio-eudaimonia)? Again, this occurs through emergence. Socio-eudaimonia, is a higher-level construct based on eudaimonia, but also takes on well-being elements related to the interaction of the individual with the social environment. The well-being element that captures such social interactions is referred to as social well-being in the well-being literature (e.g., Keyes, 1998, 2002, 2007, 2013). In sum, high levels of eudaimonia at the developmental level mediated by a process involving high social and moral development result into high levels of socio-eudaimonia at the social-ecological level; and conversely, low levels of eudaimonia mediated by a process involving low social and moral development result into low levels of socio-eudaimonia.

Conclusion

The concept of *positive balance* is consistent with much of the discussion of "Second Wave Positive Psychology" (Lomas, Hefferon, & Ivtzan, 2015; Lomas & Ivtzan, 2016). Second Wave Positive Psychology is an emerging movement within positive psychology that acknowledges the problems inherent in treating positive mental health concepts as either "positive" or "negative." As such, the movement recognizes the dialectical nature of positive mental health–a complex and dynamic interplay of positive and negative mental states. As succinctly captured by Ryff and Singer (2003, p. 272), well-being involves "inevitable dialectics between positive and negative aspects of living."

The concept of positive mental health as extracted from the positive psychology movement has been criticized because of its overemphasis on individualism and positive thinking. For example, Ehrenreich (2009) has asserted that positive psychologists preaching the concept of positive mental health, based on individualism and positive thinking and set apart from the larger culture, have overpromised the public. They overpromised to transform people's lives by merely thinking positively while ignoring what should be changed in the environment to help change people's lives. The social environment plays a significant role in the make-up of well-being. Of course, if we strictly focus on the individual without understanding how the environment affects positive mental health then there should be no call to action on the political front. The positive psychology movement implies that life coaches and therapists advise their clients and patients to change themselves by changing their thought pattern. Instead, to enhance positive mental health much can be done to change social institutions. Other critics have voiced similar concerns (e.g., Allen, 2018; Davies, 2016; Held, 2002, 2005). The concept of well-being introduced here considers many disciplinary aspects of the discourse on mental well-being—aspects from physiology, the study of emotions, cognitive science, human development, and sociology.

References

Aderem, A. (2005). Systems biology: Its practice and challenges. *Cell, 121*, 511–513.

Allen, J. (2018). *The psychology of happiness in the modern world*. New York: Springer.

Andrews, F. M., & Withey, S. B. (1976). *Social indicators of well-being: America's perception of life quality*. New York: Plenum.

Bauer, J. J. (2016). Eudaimonic growth: The development of the goods in personhood (or: Cultivating a good life story). In J. Vitterso (Ed.), *Handbook of eudaimonic well-being* (pp. 147–174). Dordrecht: Springer.

Baumeister, R. F., & Leary, M. R. (1995). The need to belong: Desire for interpersonal attachments as a fundamental human motivation. *Psychological Bulletin, 117*, 497–523.

Bremner, J. D., Randall, P., Scott, T. M., Bronen, R. A., Seibyl, J. P., Southwick, S. M., et al. (1995). MRI-based measurement of hippocampal volume in patients with combat-related posttraumatic stress disorder. *American Journal of Psychiatry, 152*, 973–981.

Bretherton, I. (1985). Attachment theory: Retrospect and prospect. *Monographs of the Society for Research in Child Development, 50*(1–2), 3–35.

Campbell, A., Converse, P. E., & Rodgers, W. L. (1976). *The quality of American life: Perspectives, evaluations, and satisfactions*. New York: Russell Sage Foundation.

Carlquist, E., Ulleberg, P., Delle Fave, A., Nafstad, H. E., & Blakar, R. M. (2017). Everyday understandings of happiness, good life, and satisfaction: Three different facets of well-being. *Applied Research in Quality of Life, 12*, 481–505.

Catalino, L. I., Algoe, S. B., & Fredrickson, B. L. (2011). Prioritizing positivity: An effective approach to pursuing happiness? *Emotion, 14*, 1155–1161.

Crommelinck, M., Feltz, B., & Goujon, P. (Eds.). (2006). *Self-organization and emergence in life sciences*. Heidelberg: Springer.

Csikszentmihalyi, M., & LeFevre, J. (1989). Optimal experience in work and leisure. *Journal of Personality and Social Psychology, 56*, 815–822.

Dambrun, M., Ricard, M., Despres, G., Drelon, E., Gibelin, E., Gilbelin, M., et al. (2012). Measuring happiness: From fluctuating happiness to authentic-durable happiness. *Frontiers in Psychology, 3*, article 16.

Davies, W. (2016). *The happiness industry: How the government and big business sold us well-being*. London, UK: Verso.

Day, R. L. (1987). Relationship between life satisfaction and consumer satisfaction. In A. C. Samli (Ed.), *Marketing and quality-of-life interface* (pp. 289–311). Westport, CT: Greenwood Press.

Deci, E. L., & Ryan, R. M. (2008). Hedonia, eudaimonia, and well-being: An introduction. *Journal of Happiness Studies, 9*, 1–11.

Delle Fave, A., Brdar, I., Freire, T., Vella-Brodrick, D., & Wissing, M. P. (2011). The eudaimonic and hedonic components of happiness: Qualitative and quantitative findings. *Social Indicators Research, 100*, 185–207.

Denson, T. F., Spanovic, M., & Miller, N. (2009). Cognitive appraisals and emotions predict cortisol and immune responses: A meta-analysis of acute laboratory social stressors and emotion inductions. *Psychological Bulletin, 135*, 823–845.

Diener, E. (1984). Subjective well-being. *Psychological Bulletin, 95*, 542–575.

Diener, E., & Emmons, R. A. (1984). The independence of positive and negative affect. *Journal of Personality and Social Psychology, 47*, 1105–1117.

Diener, E., Fujita, F., Tay, L., & Biswas-Diener, R. (2012). Purpose, mood, and pleasure in predicting satisfaction judgments. *Social Indicators Research, 105*, 333–341.

Diener, E., Suh, E. M., Lucas, R. E., & Smith, H. L. (1999). Subjective well-being: Three decades of progress. *Psychological Bulletin, 125*, 276–302.

Diener, E., Wirtz, D., Tov, W., Kim-Prieto, C., Choi, D., Oishi, S., et al. (2010). New well-being measures: Short scales to assess flourishing and positive and negative feelings. *Social Indicators Research, 97*, 143–156.

Duckworth, A. L., & Gross, J. J. (2014). Self-control and grit: Related but separable determinants of success. *Current Directions in Psychological Science, 23*, 319–325.

Ehrenreich, B. (2009). *Bright-sided: How the relentless promotion of positive thinking has undermined America*. New York: Metropolitan Books.

Forgas, J. P. (2014). On the downside of feeling good: Evidence for the motivational, cognitive, and behavioral disadvantages of positive affect. In J. Gruber & J. T. Moskowitz (Eds.), *Positive emotion: Integrating the light sides and the dark sides* (pp. 301–322). New York: Oxford University Press.

Fredrickson, B. L. (2001). The role of positive emotions in positive psychology: The broaden-and-build theory of positive emotions. *American Psychologist, 56*, 218–222.

Fredrickson, B. L. (2004). The broaden-and-build theory of positive emotions. *Philosophical Transactions of the Royal Society B: Biological Sciences, 359*(1449), 1367–1377.

Fredrickson, B. L. (2009). *Positivity: Top-notch research reveals the 3-to-1 ratio that will change your life*. New York: Three Rivers Press.

Fredrickson, B. L. (2013). Updated thinking on positivity ratios. *American Psychologist, 68*, 814–822.

Fredrickson, B. L., & Joiner, T. (2002). Positive emotions trigger upward spirals toward emotional well-being. *Psychological Science, 13*, 172–175.

Frieswijk, N., Buunk, B. P., Steverink, N., & Slaets, J. P. (2004). The effect of social comparison information on the life satisfaction of frail older persons. *Psychology and Aging, 19*, 183–198.

Gallagher, M. W., Lopez, S. J., & Preacher, K. J. (2009). The hierarchical structure of well-being. *Journal of Personality, 77*, 1025–1049.

Gilbertson, M. W., Shenton, M. E., Ciszewski, A., Kasai, K., Lasko, N. B., Orr, S. P., et al. (2002). Smaller hippocampal volume predicts pathologic vulnerability to psychological trauma. *Nature Neuroscience, 5*, 1242–1247.

Headey, B., Holmstrom, E., & Wearing, A. (1984). Well-being and ill-being: Different dimensions. *Social Indicators Research, 14*, 115–139.

Held, B. S. (2002). The tyranny of the positive attitude in America: Observation and speculation. *Journal of Clinical Psychology, 58*, 965–992.

Held, B. S. (2005). The "virtues" of positive psychology. *Journal of Theoretical and Philosophical Psychology, 25*, 1–34.

Ho, S. S. M., & Chan, R. S. Y. (2009). Social harmony in Hong Kong: Level, determinants, and policy implications. *Social Indicators Research, 91*, 37–58.

Hostinar, C. E., & Gunnar, M. R. (2013). Future directions in the study of social relationships as regulators of the HPA axis across development. *Journal of Clinical Child and Adolescent Psychology, 42*, 564–575.

Huta, V., & Waterman, A. S. (2014). Eudaimonia and its distinction from hedonia: Developing a classification and terminology for understanding conceptual and operational definitions. *Journal of Happiness Studies, 15*, 1425–1456.

Jackson, P. A., Sirgy, M. J., & Medley, G. D. (2018). The neurobiology of well-being. In N. R. Silton (Ed.), *Scientific concepts behind happiness, kindness and empathy in contemporary society* (pp. 135–155). Hershey, PA: IGI Global.

Jahoda, M. (1958). *Current concepts of positive mental health*. New York: Basic Books.

Joseph, S., & Wood, A. (2010). Assessment of positive functioning in clinical psychology: Theoretical and practical issues. *Clinical Psychology Review, 30*, 830–838.

Joshanloo, M. (2016). Revisiting the empirical distinction between hedonic and eudaimonic aspects of well-being using exploratory structural equation modeling. *Journal of Happiness Studies, 17*, 2023–2036.

Joshanloo, M., Bobowick, M., & Basabe, N. (2016). Factor structure of mental well-being: Contributions of exploratory structural equation modeling. *Personality and Individual Differences, 102*, 107–110.

Joshanloo, M., & Weijers, D. (2014). Aversion to happiness across cultures: A review of where and why people are averse to happiness. *Journal of Happiness Studies, 15*, 717–735.

Kahneman, D., Diener, E., & Schwarz, N. (1999). Preface. In D. Kahneman, E. Diener, & N. Schwarz (Eds.), *Well-being: The foundations of a hedonic psychology* (pp. 9–12). New York: Russell Sage Foundation.

Keyes, C. L. M. (1998). Social well-being. *Social Psychology Quarterly, 61*, 121–140.

Keyes, C. L. M. (2002). The mental health continuum: From languishing to flourishing in life. *Journal of Health and Social Behavior, 43*, 207–222.

Keyes, C. L. M. (2003). Complete mental health: An agenda for the 21st century. In C. L. M. Keyes & J. Haidt (Eds.), *Flourishing: Positive psychology and the life well-lived* (pp. 293–312). Washington, DC: American Psychological Association.

Keyes, C. L. M. (2007). Promoting and protecting mental health as flourishing: A complementary strategy for improving national mental health. *American Psychologist, 62*, 95–108.

Keyes, C. L. M. (Ed.). (2013). *Mental well-being: International contributions to the study of positive mental health*. Dordrecht: Springer.

Keyes, C. L. M., & Lopez, S. J. (2002). Toward a science of mental health: Positive directions in diagnosis and interventions. In C. R. Snyder & S. J. Lopez (Eds.), *The handbook of positive psychology* (pp. 45–59). New York: Oxford University Press.

Keyes, C. L., Shmotkin, D., & Ryff, C. D. (2002). Optimizing well-being: The empirical encounter of two traditions. *Journal of Personality and Social Psychology, 82*, 1007–1022.

Keyes, C. L. M., & Waterman, M. B. (2003). Dimensions of well-being and mental health in adulthood. In M. Bornstein, L. Davidson, C. L. M. Keyes, & K. A. Moore (Eds.), *Well-being: Positive development throughout the life course* (pp. 481–501). Mahwah, NJ: Erlbaum.

Lee, W.-S., & Oguzoglu, U. (2004). Well-being and ill-being: A bivariate panel data analysis. A Discussion Paper. http://papers.ssrn.com/sol3/papers.cfm?abstract_id=1029914

Lee, D.-J., & Sirgy, M. J. (2018). What do people do to achieve work-life balance? A formative conceptualization to help develop a metric for large-scale quality-of-life surveys. *Social Indicators Research, 138*, 771–791.

Lomas, T., Hefferon, K., & Ivtzan, I. (2015). The LIFE model: A meta-theoretical conceptual map for applied positive psychology. *Journal of Happiness Studies, 16*, 1347–1364.

Lomas, T., & Ivtzan, I. (2016). Second wave positive psychology: Exploring the positive-negative dialectics of wellbeing. *Journal of Happiness Studies, 17*, 1753–1768.

Lovallo, W. R. (2016). *Stress & health: Biological and psychological interactions*. Thousand Oaks, CA: Sage Publications.

McEwen, B. S., & Wingfield, J. C. (2003). The concept of allostasis in biology and biomedicine. *Hormones and Behavior, 43*, 2–15.

Meadow, H. L., Mentzer, J. J., Rahtz, D. R., & Sirgy, M. J. (1992). A life satisfaction measure based on judgment theory. *Social Indicators Research, 26*, 23–59.

Michalos, A. C. (1985). Multiple discrepancies theory (MDT). *Social Indicators Research, 16*, 347–413.

Michalos, A. C. (1986). An application of Multiple Discrepancies Theory (MDT) to seniors. *Social Indicators Research, 18*, 349–373.

Michalos, A. C., Hatch, P. M., Hemingway, D., Lavallee, L., Hogan, A., & Christensen, B. (2007). Health and quality of life of older people, a replication after six years. *Social Indicators Research, 84*, 127–158.

Morling, B., & Fiske, S. T. (1999). Defining and measuring harmony control. *Journal of Research in Personality, 33*, 379–414.

Munoz Sastre, M. T. (1998). Lay conceptions of well-being and rules used in well-being judgements among young, middle-aged, and elderly adults. *Social Indicators Research, 47*, 203–231.

Pavot, W., & Diener, E. (1993). Review of the satisfaction with life scale. *Psychological Assessment, 5*, 164–172.

Pavot, W., Diener, E., & Suh, E. (1998). The temporal satisfaction with life scale. *Journal of Personality Assessment, 70*, 340–354.

Pressman, S. D., & Cohen, S. (2005). Does positive affect influence health? *Psychological Bulletin, 131*, 925–971.

Robitschek, C., & Keyes, C. L. M. (2009). Keyes's model of mental health with personal growth initiative as a parsimonious predictor. *Journal of Counseling Psychology, 56*, 321–329.

Rockwood, K., Hogan, D. B., & MacKnight, C. (2000). Conceptualisation and measurement of frailty in elderly people. *Drugs & Aging, 17*, 295–302.

Rowe, C. J., & Broadie, S. (Eds.). (2002). *Nicomachean ethics*. USA: Oxford University Press.

Ryan, R. M., & Deci, E. L. (2000). Self-determination theory and the facilitation of intrinsic motivation, social development and well-being. *American Psychologist, 55*, 68–78.

Ryan, R. M., Huta, V., & Deci, E. L. (2008). Living well: A self-determination theory perspective on eudaimonia. *Journal of Happiness Studies, 9*, 139–170.

Ryan, R. M., & Martela, F. (2016). Eudaimonia as a way of living: Connecting Aristotle with self-determination theory. In J. Vitterso (Ed.), *Handbook of eudaimonic well-being* (pp. 109–122). Dordrecht: Springer.

Ryff, C. D. (1989). Happiness is everything, or is it? Explorations on the meaning of psychological well-being. *Journal of Personality and Social Psychology, 57*, 1069–1081.

Ryff, C. D., & Singer, B. (2003). Ironies of the human condition: Well-being and health on the way to mortality. In L. G. Aspinwall & U. M. Staudinger (Eds.), *A psychology of human strengths* (pp. 271–287). Washington, DC: American Psychological Association.

Schwartz, B. (2015). *Why we work*. New York: Simon & Schuster.

Schwartz, B., & Wrzesniewski, A. (2016). Internal motivation, instrumental motivation, and eudaimonia. In J. Vitterso (Ed.), *Handbook of eudaimonic well-being* (pp. 123–134). Dordrecht: Springer.

Shapiro, A., & Keyes, C. L. M. (2008). Marital status and social well-being: Are the married always better off? *Social Indicators Research, 88*, 329–346.

Sirgy, M. J. (2012). *The psychology of quality of life: Hedonic well-being, life satisfaction, and eudaimonia*. Dordrecht: Springer.

Sirgy, M. J. (2019). Positive balance: A hierarchical perspective of positive mental health. *Quality of Life Research, 28*(7), 1921–1930.

Sirgy, M. J., Cole, D., Kosenko, R., Meadow, H. L., Rahtz, R. D., Cicic, M., et al. (1995). Judgment-type life satisfaction measure: Further validation. *Social Indicators Research, 34*, 237–259.

Sirgy, M. J., & Lee, D.-J. (2016). Work-life balance: A quality-of-life model. *Applied Research in Quality of Life, 11*, 1059–1082.

Sirgy, M. J., & Lee, D.-J. (2018a). Work-life balance: An integrative review. *Applied Research in Quality of Life, 13*, 229–254.

Sirgy, M. J., & Lee, D.-J. (2018b). The psychology of life balance. In E. Diener, S. Oishi, & L. Tay (Eds.), *e-Handbook of subjective well-being*. NobaScholar.

Sirgy, M. J., & Wu, J. (2009). The pleasant life, the engaged life, and the meaningful life: What about the balanced life? *Journal of Happiness Studies, 10*, 183–196.

Solé, R. V., Ferrer-Cancho, R., Montoya, J. M., & Valverde, S. (2002). Selection, tinkering, and emergence in complex networks. *Complexity, 8*, 20–33.

Spinelli, S., Schwandt, M. L., Lindell, S. G., Heilig, M., Suomi, S. J., Higley, J. D., et al. (2012). The serotonin transporter gene linked polymorphic region is associated with the behavioral response to repeated stress exposure in infant rhesus macaques. *Developmental and Psychopathology, 24*, 157–165.

Sterling, P., & Eyer, J. (1988). Allostasis: A new paradigm to explain arousal pathology. In S. Fisher & J. Reason (Eds.), *Handbook of life stress, cognition, and health* (pp. 629–649). New York, NY: Wiley.

Suh, E., Diener, E., Oishi, S., & Triandis, H. C. (1998). The shifting basis of life satisfaction judgments across cultures: Emotions versus norms. *Journal of Personality and Social Psychology, 74*, 482–495.

Vitterso, J. (Ed.). (2016). *Handbook of eudaimonic well-being*. Dordrecht: Springer.

Waterman, A. S. (1993). Two conceptions of happiness: Contrasts of personal expressiveness (eudaimonia) and hedonic enjoyment. *Journal of Personality and Social Psychology, 64*, 678–691.

Wolfer, R., & Scheithauer, H. (2013). Ostracism in childhood and adolescence: Emotional, cognitive, and behavioral effects of social exclusion. *Social Influence, 8*, 1–20.

Chapter 2
Positive Balance at the Physiological Level: Positive and Negative Neurotransmitters

Introduction

Understanding the physiological and neurological features of spiritual experiences should not be interpreted as an attempt to discredit their reality or explain them away. Rather, it demonstrates their physical existence as a fundamental, shared part of human nature. Spiritual experiences cannot be considered irrational, since we have seen that, given their physiological basis, experiencers' descriptions of them are perfectly rational... All human perceptions of material reality can ultimately be documented as chemical reactions in our neurobiology; all our sensations, thoughts, and memories are ultimately reducible to chemistry, yet we feel no need to deny the existence of the material world; it is not less real because our perceptions of it are biologically based... It is not rational to assume that the spiritual reality of core experiences is any less real than the more scientifically documentable material reality.—Sabina Magliocco, *Witching Culture: Folklore and Neo-Paganism in America* (https://www.goodreads.com/work/quotes/851274-witching-culture-folklore-and-neo-paganism-in-america-contemporary-eth)

In Chap. 1, I offered a definition of positive mental health from a physiological perspective capturing what I believe as a state of positive balance. To reiterate, the positive balance definition of positive mental health at the physiological level is as follows: *Positive mental health is a state of mind in which is the individual experiences a preponderance of neurochemicals related to rewards (e.g., dopamine, serotonin, and oxytocin) relative to neurochemicals related to stress (e.g., cortisol).* In this chapter, I will discuss the research that supports this view of positive mental health. I will refer to two research programs, namely the neurobiology of hedonic well-being and the stress response system. I briefly discussed these two programs of research in Chap. 1 but delve in greater detail in this chapter. See the highlighted part in Table 2.1 to help focus the discussion.

© Springer Nature Switzerland AG 2020
M. J. Sirgy, *Positive Balance*, Social Indicators Research Series 80,
https://doi.org/10.1007/978-3-030-40289-1_2

Table 2.1 Positive mental health defined at the physiological level

Level of analysis	Positive balance as positive mental health	Programs of research	Emergence
Positive mental health defined at a physiological level = **positive and negative neurotransmitters**	Individuals experiencing a preponderance of neurochemicals related to positive emotions (dopamine, serotonin, oxytocin) relative to neurochemicals related to negative emotions (cortisol)	Stress response system); neurobiology of happiness)	
Positive mental health defined at an emotional level = **positive/negative affect or hedonic well-being (positive/negative neurotransmitters + cognitive appraisals)**	Individuals experiencing a preponderance of positive emotions (happiness, joy, serenity, contentment, etc.) relative to negative emotions (anger, sadness, jealousy, envy, depression, etc.)	Positive versus negative affect; broaden and build theory; flow	Positive neurochemicals (dopamine, serotonin, and oxytocin) at the physiological level mediated by a process of cognitive appraisal (positive frame) result into positive affect (happiness, joy, contentment, etc.) at the emotional level; and conversely, negative neurochemicals (cortisol) mediated by a process of cognitive appraisal (negative frame) result into negative affect (anger, sadness, jealousy, envy, depression, etc.)
Positive mental health defined at a cognitive level = **domain satisfaction (positive/negative affect + domain segmentation)**	Individuals experiencing a preponderance of domain satisfaction (satisfaction in salient and multiple life domains such as family life, work life, social life, etc.) relative to dissatisfaction in other life domains	Principle of satisfaction limits; principle of the full spectrum of human developmental needs; principle of diminishing satisfaction	Positive affect (happiness, joy, contentment, etc.) at the emotional level mediated by a process of domain segmentation result into domain satisfaction (satisfied with work life, social life, family life, etc.); and conversely, negative affect (anger, sadness, jealousy, envy, depression, etc.) mediated by a process of domain segmentation result into domain dissatisfaction (dissatisfied with work life, social life, family life, etc.)
Positive mental health defined at a meta-cognitive level = **life satisfaction (domain satisfaction + bottom-up process)**	Individuals experiencing a preponderance of positive evaluations about one's life using certain standards of comparison (satisfaction with one's life compared to one's past life, the life of family members, the life of associates at work, the life of others in the same social circles, etc.) relative to negative evaluations about one's life using similar or other standards of comparison	Multiple discrepancies theory; congruity life satisfaction; temporal life satisfaction; social comparison; frequency of positive affect; homeostatically protected mood	Domain satisfaction (satisfied with work life, social life, family life, etc.) at the cognitive level mediated by a bottom-up process at the meta-cognitive level result in life satisfaction; and conversely. domain dissatisfaction (dissatisfied with work life, social life, family life, etc.) mediated by a bottom-up process result in life dissatisfaction

(continued)

Table 2.1 (continued)

Positive mental health defined at a developmental level = **eudaimonia (life satisfaction + personal growth)**	Individuals experiencing a preponderance of positive psychological traits (self-acceptance, personal growth, purpose in life, environmental mastery, autonomy, positive relations with others, etc.) relative to negative psychological traits (pessimism, hopelessness, depressive disorder, neuroticism, impulsiveness, etc.)	Hedonic versus eudaimonic happiness; virtue ethics and character strengths; self-determination theory; personal expressiveness; psychological well-being; purpose and meaning in life; flourishing; orientations to happiness; resilience; and satisfaction of the full spectrum of human needs	Life satisfaction at the meta-cognitive level mediated by a process involving high personal growth result in high levels of eudaimonia at the developmental level; and conversely, life dissatisfaction mediated by a process involving low personal growth result into low levels of eudaimonia
Positive mental health defined at a social-ecological level = **socio-eudaimonia (eudaimonia + social & moral development)**	Individuals experiencing a preponderance of social resources (social acceptance, social actualization, social contribution, social integration, social harmony, social belonginess, social attachment, familial attachment, etc.) relative to social constraints (social alienation, social discord, social exclusion, ostracism, etc.)	Social well-being, social harmony need to belong, attachment theory; social exclusion and ostracism	High levels of eudaimonia at the developmental level mediated by a process involving high social and moral development result into high levels of socio-eudaimonia at the social-ecological level; and conversely, low levels of eudaimonia mediated by a process involving low social and moral development result into low levels of socio-eudaimonia

Programs of Research Supporting the Positive Balance Definition

In the sections below I will discuss two major programs of research in psychophysiology supporting the definition of positive mental health at the physiological level. These are: the neurobiology of hedonic well-being and the stress response system and cortisol.

The Neurobiology of Hedonic Well-Being[1]

Research in neuroscience has identified the major neurotransmitters implicated in positive affect: dopamine, serotonin, and oxytocin. In contrast, cortisol is associated

---

[1]This section is adapted partly from Jackson, Sirgy, and Medley (2018).

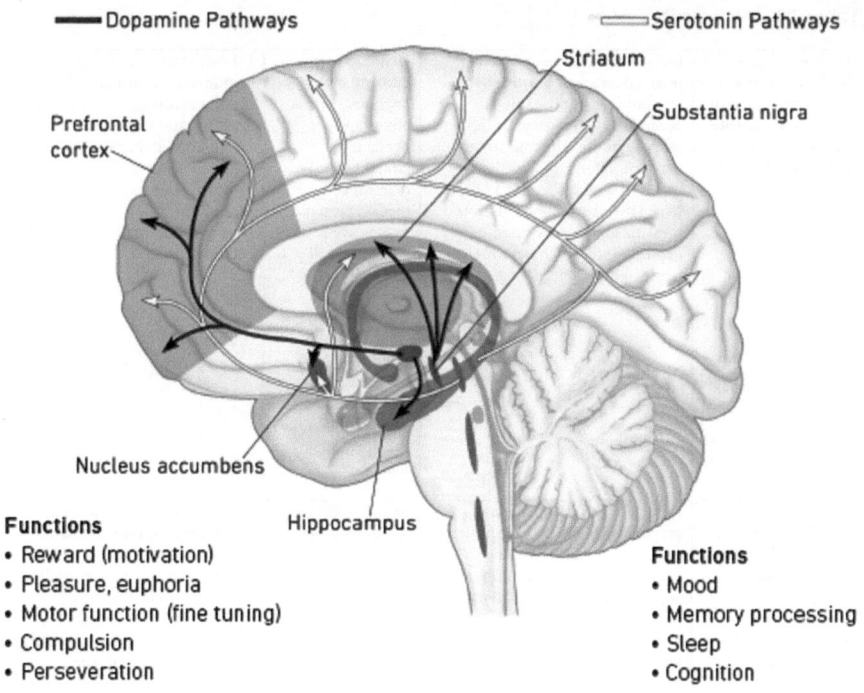

Fig. 2.1 Dopamine and serotonin pathways. Source: National Institutes of Health, U.S. Department of Health and Human Services

with negative affect (see literature review by Jackson, Sirgy, & Medley, 2018). *Dopamine* plays a significant role in positive affect. It is the primary neurotransmitter operating in the brain reward system. All pleasurable activities (e.g., engaging in sexual intercourse, listening to music, eating and drinking when feeling hungry) are associated with the influx of dopamine. Reduced levels of *serotonin* are associated with negative mood, anxiety, and depression (see Fig. 2.1 for dopamine and serotonin pathways in the brain). *Oxytocin* is associated with maternal feelings as in childbirth and lactation, mother-infant bonding, and prosocial behavior. Allow me to be more specific. The reader should be in a better position to appreciate the role of these neurotransmitters in well-being through a discussion of the reward center and drugs and neurotransmitters.

The Reward Center and Well-Being What is the mechanism of action that produces pleasant emotions that result in hedonic well-being? The mechanism involves brain centers that reflect what neuroscientists refer to as "the reward system" (Wise, 1996). The seminal study demonstrating the presence of the reward circuit involved rats that pressed a bar to administer a brief burst of electrical stimulation to specific sites in their brains (Olds & Milner, 1954). Said behavior had no value to their survival (i.e., food) nor to that of the species (i.e., sex), but resulted in compulsive repetition of bar pressing. This phenomenon has been referred to as "intracranial self-stimulation" or "brain-stimulation reward" (Wise, 1996).

Research investigating intracranial self-stimulation has identified several brain sites that are involved in the reward system. Some regions stand out more than others such as the ventral tegmental area, or VTA, and the medial forebrain bundle. Stimulation of these regions activates fibers that form the ascending pathways from dopamine-producing cells of the VTA that project to the nucleus accumbens (NAc), the amygdala, the hippocampus, and the prefrontal cortex (Advokat, Comaty, & Julien, 2014; Kolb & Whishaw, 2014; Rickard & Vella-Brodrick, 2014). This system, referred to as the mesolimbic dopamine pathway, plays a crucial role in rewards. Drugs of abuse activate this reward system either directly (e.g., cocaine) or indirectly (e.g., opium). Much evidence shows that increases in dopamine (a neurotransmitter) in this pathway are directly involved with positive affect—feelings of pleasure and even euphoria.

The mesolimbic system shows a marked increase of dopamine when animals are engaged in intracranial self-stimulation (Olds & Milner, 1954). The same system shows a marked increase of dopamine when animals engage in rewarding behaviors (e.g., feeding and copulation). The reward system also shows a marked increase in dopamine with all drugs taken for pleasure, such as amphetamines, opiates, barbiturates, alcohol, THC, PCP, MDMA, nicotine, and even caffeine (Kolb & Whishaw, 2014, p. 438). Other addictions, such as compulsive gambling, pathological overeating, and sexual addiction, have also been strongly correlated with changes in the VTA-NAc dopamine system (Nestler, 2005). Chronic dopamine activation diminishes endogenous dopamine release and causes down-regulation of dopamine receptors which is a major aspect of drug tolerance (Volkow et al., 2005). Fewer dopamine receptors creates a "reward deficiency syndrome" that accounts for addicts' lowered responsiveness to natural rewards and predisposes addicts to seek out drugs to experience even normal levels of pleasure.

Other neurons interact with the dopamine-producing neurons in the VTA, and other neurotransmitters are involved in the increase of dopamine in the system as well. The endogenous opioid system (EOS) is one of the principal modulators of the mesolimbic dopaminergic reward circuitry (Mathew & Paulose, 2011). The use of acupuncture has been linked to the enhancement of endogenous opiates, resulting in pain relief from multiple disorders, surgeries, and diseases (Patil et al., 2016). The "runner's high" is an example of intense pleasure following the release of endogenous opiates (endorphins) during prolonged vigorous exercise (Gianoulakis, 2001). When observing individuals with borderline personality disorder (BPD), these individuals will go to any means to experience pleasure, regardless of the harmful effects that may accompany it, such as using whips to cause heavy bleeding to reach a heightened state of ecstasy (Gratz & Gunderson, 2006). This suggests a dysregulation in the EOS of individuals with BPD.

Panksepp (2005) has argued that the brain reward center is the motivating force underlying growth needs or higher order needs *a la* Maslow (cf. Silton, Flannelly, Flannelly, & Galek, 2011). Specific areas of the limbic system (i.e., the reward center) may help actualize a diversity of internal wants and desires, thus motivating the individual to satisfy growth needs that lead to positive affect. On the other hand, the person that seeks to increase hedonic well-being by using drugs regularly will experience lower levels of hedonic well-being because of the tolerance that develops. The reasons are threefold and due largely to the changes in the reward center: (1) the reduction in dopamine and dopamine receptors in the VTA means that the person will feel less pleasure in general when the drug is not on board, and (2) they will need greater amounts of the drug to experience the original level of euphoria the drug produced, and (3) to satisfy the craving that results and the need for the euphoric effect, the person will spend greater time and resources engaging in drug seeking behavior, time and resources needed to maintain an acceptable level of positive affect.

In sum, the brain center responsible for hedonic well-being reflects what neuroscientists refer to as the reward system. The reward system involves several regions in the brain. Stimulation of these regions activates pathways from the VTA that project to the NAc, the amygdala, the hippocampus, and the prefrontal cortex (i.e., the mesolimbic dopamine pathway). Increases in dopamine in this circuit produce feelings of pleasure or positive affect and lower levels of cortisol. The mesolimbic system is characterized by marked increases in dopamine with all drugs taken for pleasure, such as amphetamines, opiates, barbiturates, alcohol, THC, PCP, MDMA, nicotine, caffeine, and even compulsive gambling, pathological overeating, and sexual addiction. Other systems interact with the mesolimbic system such as the endogenous opioid system. Individuals seeking to increase hedonic well-being through drug use are likely to experience lower levels of positive affect over time because of the adverse effects of drug tolerance.

Drugs, Neurotransmitters, and Hedonic Well-Being Throughout the history of humanity, people have used drugs of all types to make them feel happy and numb the pain of life's adversities. Probably the most common drug is alcohol. Other drugs include opium (derivatives of opium include morphine and heroin), cocaine, amphetamines, benzodiazepines, and cannabis (THC). These, and many other drugs, stimulate the reward system and produce euphoria in the user, which makes these drugs key candidates for abuse.

Cocaine (a potent psychostimulant) can dramatically induce the release of dopamine (as well as norepinephrine, epinephrine, and serotonin). The net effect is heightened alertness, euphoria, lowered fatigue, decreased boredom, depressed appetite, and insomnia (Advokat, Comaty, & Julien, 2014). In 1884, Freud recommended using cocaine to alleviate depression and chronic fatigue. However, the rebound symptoms (once the drug leaves the system) are fatigue and depression (McKim & Hancock, 2013) making the therapeutic use of cocaine for depression ill advised.

Looby and Earleywine (2007) compared a large sample of people that had never used methamphetamine to a group that had used it at least once in the past year. They found that methamphetamine use decreased hedonic well-being. The study was also predictive of feeling more depressed and apathetic, less happy and having lower levels of satisfaction with life. This could mean that unhappy people seek out psychostimulants to self-medicate, or it could indicate that using methamphetamine produces depression, symptoms of which have been shown to be increased in methamphetamine users in other studies (e.g., Dyer & Cruickshank, 2005). While acute use may produce momentary hedonia, it has long-term detrimental effects on other forms of well-being (life satisfaction and eudaimonia).

Opiates (morphine, codeine, and heroin) have euphoric effects. In small doses opiates decrease anxiety and reduce pain; higher doses can produce euphoria. The brain and body make their own opiate-like chemicals, commonly referred to as "endorphins" (endogenous morphine-like peptides). Endorphins control pain by stopping the flow of pain signals to the brain. Engaging in physical activities such as distance running could produce an "endorphin high."

Clearly, drugs that act on the reward system in the brain influence hedonic well-being (i.e., short-term positive and negative affect). Research has also shown drugs such as opiates may activate both dopaminergic and nondopaminergic systems (e.g., Spanagel & Weiss, 1999). Such findings led to the development of the *incentive-sensitization theory of addiction* (Robinson & Berridge, 1993, 2003). This theory asserts that rewards involve two separate systems: "wanting" (which may be viewed as an incentive) and "liking" (which can be viewed as evaluation of the pleasant sensation). For example, a person may feel the desire to eat chocolate ("wanting"), and he may experience a pleasant sensation having eaten the chocolate ("liking"). The dopamine system seems to be related to both the "wanting" and "liking" components, whereas the "liking" component may also involve opioid and GABA (an inhibitory neurotransmitter) systems.

Another theory explains the role of dopamine in learning. Specifically, the dopamine system responds to the "unpredictability of rewards" (Berns, McClure, Pagnoni, & Montague, 2001) or errors in prediction (Schultz, 2002). That is, learning occurs when the reward is better or worse than expected. Learning does not occur when the reward matches expectations. Dopamine release is concomitant with learning. This learning is evidenced in brain plasticity involving significant neuronal changes—increased dendritic length and complexity in the nucleus accumbens and prefrontal cortex, as well as activity increases in areas involved in learning such as the hippocampus (e.g., Robinson & Berridge, 2001). Given the dopamine release in situations when expectations are negatively disconfirmed (worse than expectations), dissatisfaction may follow, and of course dissatisfaction is reflective of negative affect. Negative affect cannot be construed as "reward." Hence, neuroscientists now feel more comfortable using the term "reinforcer" rather than "reward." In other words, dopamine plays a crucial role in the "reinforcement" system (i.e., learning), as well as in the "reward" system.[2] In addition, large and fast increases in dopamine, such as those triggered by drugs, are associated with phasic

---

[2]It should be noted that the current level of hedonic well-being experienced by an individual is likely to moderate the effects of euphoric drugs, such as pain killers or psychostimulants, as well. This phenomenon is commonly known as the "Law of Initial Value" (Wilder, 1958). Wilder's law states that a change, such as that produced by a drug, cannot affect the person's mood or cognitive state beyond their capability for change. In addition, the effect of the drug depends on the user's initial state. If the person is close to their maximum state for the effect in question, then little change will occur; however, if they are quite distant then the greater the potential effect. For example, a person who is currently in a negative mood state (i.e., experiencing anxiety, pain, or melancholy) may experience euphoria when given small doses of morphine. In contrast, a similar dose of morphine given to a happy person may have little effect or even induce anxiety and fear (Wenk, 2009, p. 20).

dopamine firing in the brain, which conveys information about saliency as well as reward (Schultz, 2010). Therefore, when a person expects a certain euphoric high from taking a drug, but the euphoria is lower because tolerance has developed, they will experience negative affect. This may contribute to the decreases in life satisfaction observed in those with substance-use disorder.

Based on the research related to drug dependence (e.g., Kalivas & Volkow, 2005; Kalivas, Peters, & Knackstedt, 2006; Volkow et al., 2005), the following theoretical notions concerning well-being can be extrapolated:

1. Humans possess a reward circuit that is activated by both drug and non-drug rewards. The most well-known reward circuit involves stimulation of neurons in the ventral tegmental area which project to and cause release of dopamine in the nucleus accumbens, amygdala, and prefrontal cortex. This produces subjective feelings of pleasure.
2. Thus, dopamine underlies the reward experience and promotes learning through brain plasticity. The projections, over time, facilitate brain changes (at the neuronal level) promoting learned associations with those behaviors perceived to have led to positive affect or the reduction of negative affect, as well as progressive tolerance to the substance, ultimately resulting in less pleasure. With repeated exposure to the drug, there is a transition such that activation begins to occur more in the dorsal striatum (the caudate nucleus) as opposed to the nucleus accumbens. This is thought to underlie habit learning, in which drug taking switches from a reward-motivated behavior to a behavior that is automatic, habitual, and even compulsive. This results in negative emotionality, but also higher drug craving (see Volkow et al., 2014 on marijuana abusers).
3. Although dopamine release in the nucleus accumbens is important for the association between the behavior and the reward to be established, repeated behaviors (i.e., habits) cause recruitment of the frontal cortex and involves glutaminergic efferents to the nucleus accumbens, amygdala, and hippocampus. Kasanetz et al. (2010) found that rats developing an addiction to cocaine via self-administration showed permanent impairments in long-term-depression in the nucleus accumbens, whereas those rats exhibiting controlled drug intake were able to recover this form of neural plasticity.
4. Habits then persist as a result of enduring cellular changes in glutamate neurons in the frontal cortex. These glutaminergic projections from the frontal cortex to the nucleus accumbens are involved in motivating the individual to maintain his/her habits. Interference with the glutamate pathway impairs the ability of the prefrontal cortex to mediate response inhibition and impulse control (one consequence of chronic drug use). There are increases in prefrontal cortex activity in response to the drug itself or to cues associated with drug use (e.g., Wang et al., 1999). Volkow et al. (2005) showed an increase in metabolic activity in the orbitofrontal cortex, anterior cingulate cortex, and the dorsal striatum with drug craving as well. As a result, the drug-addicted person cannot control the craving, the impulse to take the drug, or even to avoid seeking out the drug.

5. As such, the drug-addicted person cannot control the impulse to take the drug or even to avoid seeking out the drug. Drug-addicted individuals show an enhanced motivation to procure drugs; they will go to extremes to obtain drugs despite the adverse consequences. The drug seeking and drug taking motivational drives consume much time, energy, and resources undermining long-term hedonic well-being.

In sum, drugs of abuse provide us with a window to identify neurotransmitters and brain systems involved in hedonic well-being. These drugs stimulate the reward system and produce short-lived positive affect (as well as reduce negative affect). In the long-term, these same drugs undermine feelings of well-being via multiple mechanisms. The neurotransmitters involved with these drugs include dopamine, serotonin, and cortisol, which are discussed next.

Neurochemicals Related to Hedonic Well-Being With or without drugs, the preponderance of the evidence from neuroscience shows the major neurotransmitters implicated in positive affect include dopamine, serotonin, and oxytocin, with cortisol being implicated in negative affect (Advokat, Comaty, & Julien, 2014). Discussion of these neurotransmitters in relation to hedonic well-being follows.

With respect to dopamine, much evidence from psychopharmacology suggests dopamine has a direct role in the experience of positive affect because it is the primary neurotransmitter for the reward system in the brain. Most activities people engage in for pleasure (e.g., eating, drinking, having sex, listening to music) influences dopamine neurons, specifically the release of dopamine in the NAc, which then projects up to the frontal lobes (Advokat, Comaty, & Julien, 2014). The net effect is not only feelings of euphoria but also arousal and quick thinking. Wenk (2009) uses the analogy of the gas pedal and race car to explain the adaptive function of dopamine. The brain is like the race car and dopamine is like the gas pedal. The brain feels euphoria when the gas pedal is pushed, one result of which is quick thinking. The forces of evolution have shaped the brain to enjoy working fast; the faster the better. Creatures that work faster and better are likely to survive and pass this trait to the next generation.

Studies focusing on dopamine have shown maternal separation leads to a lower density of neurotransmitter sites for dopamine (e.g., Brake, Zhang, Diorio, Meaney, & Gratton, 2004). Dopamine and norepinephrine work together to allow the individual to experience positive affect. An insufficient amount of norepinephrine leads to poor concentration, restlessness, and irritability (Mathew & Paulose, 2011).

Neurons that produce and release serotonin are in the brainstem but project throughout the brain (Kolb & Whishaw, 2014). Serotonin is involved in wakefulness and modulates many psychological processes including sexual activity, aggression, sleep and body temperature. Serotonin is also implicated in the regulation of mood, anxiety, hostility, and depression. Low levels of serotonin may be the underlying cause of depression and aggressive actions (Coccaro & Kavoussi, 1997). Peirson and Heuchert (2000) found that higher levels of platelet $5\text{-}HT_2$ receptors, corresponding to lower levels of serotonin (5-HT), were significantly correlated with depressed mood in college students. Although Peirson and Heuchert's participants were not diagnosed as depressed, the authors noted that clinically depressed patients also showed this effect in several other studies. Williams et al. (2006) found that whole-blood levels of serotonin were positively correlated with positive affect using the PANAS scale, but not with negative affect. A two-way interaction between serotonin synthesis and mood is also a possibility. Meaning that while mood may be influenced by serotonin level, it may also be true that the opposite occurs–serotonin level may be influenced by mood (Mathew & Paulose, 2011).

Turning to oxytocin, research has shown this hormone to be associated with childbirth and lactation, mother-infant bonding (Kendrick, 2004), stress, and the regulation of social behavior (i.e., Elkins, 2016). Early life experiences, such as child abuse or any childhood trauma, was negatively correlated with oxytocin levels, suggesting those early experiences can cause social deficits in the future. One study confirmed the use of oxytocin as a buffer against stress in pregnant women and showed it protected women who were of high stress from developing depressive symptoms, which, in turn, may have increased sensitive maternal behavior (Zelkowitz et al., 2014). Oxytocin has also been found to reduce symptoms related to alcohol withdrawal (Pedersen et al., 2013) and cannabis craving. The use of cannabis has been linked to stress, and a study involving marijuana-dependent individuals supported this idea. McRae-Clark, Baker, Maria, and Brady (2013) assessed a baseline using the Marijuana Craving Questionnaire (MCQ). The individuals were then administered oxytocin or a placebo prior to a psychosocial stress task. Intensity of craving was assessed immediately after the task and 5-, 35-, and 60-min post task. The overall results showed a significant reduction in craving of marijuana in response to the stressor in the group that was administered oxytocin. Another observation from the study was a lower anxiety response in the oxytocin group versus the placebo group (McRae-Clark et al., 2013). Oxytocin is also released during sexual orgasm (Huppert, 2009) and while experiencing feelings of trust (Kosfeld, Heinrichs, Zak, Fischbacher, & Fehr, 2005).

With respect to cortisol, studies have shown that exposure to stressors activates the hypothalamic-pituitary adrenal (HPA) axis and results in increased secretion of the stress hormone cortisol. Individual differences in emotional style (positivity versus negativity) modulate stress-induced elevations in cortisol (e.g., Jacobs et al., 2007; Polk, Skoner, Kirschbaum, Cohen, & Doyle, 2005; Pruessner, Hellhammer, & Kirschbaum, 1999; Smyth et al., 1998). Pressman and Cohen (2005) conducted a meta-analytic study establishing an association between trait positive affect and reduced release of stress hormones (e.g., cortisol, epinephrine and norepinephrine). In aversive situations, the amygdala sends signals to the HPA axis causing cortisol to be released from the adrenal glands. As such, people with a positive affective disposition tend to have lower basal cortisol levels compared to those with a negative affective disposition.

Another method that may aid in reducing stress, which also inhibits excessive cortisol secretion, is prefrontal transcranial Direct Current Stimulation (tDCS). It involves the placement of two macro-electrodes on the skull in certain brain regions and sending a weak current between them. Austin et al. (2016) used the F3 and F4 brain regions, and applied it to healthy, early adult females to observe if there was a difference in psychological distress after tDCS. Typically, the F3 and F4 regions are used in the treatment of depression. The results yielded significantly less psychological distress from daily stressors in the participants and a decrease in negative mood states (Austin et al., 2016; Siever, 2015). The Petrocchi et al. (2017) study involved only anodal stimulation, which is related to an increase in neuronal excitability and is followed by a decrease in GABA. They sought to find a correlation between heart rate variability and positive emotion in healthy individuals. This study placed an electrode on the left temporal lobe only. Researchers found that one session of tDCS increased heart rate variability, and in return, this stimulation triggered soothing positive affect, which was associated with feelings of peacefulness, contentment, and well-being. Their study provided support for the effectiveness of tDCS on depression and other psychopathological conditions (Petrocchi et al., 2017; Stagg et al., 2009).

In sum, much of the evidence shows that the major neurotransmitters implicated in positive affect include dopamine, serotonin, and oxytocin. Cortisol, on the other hand, is implicated in negative affect.

The Stress Response System and Cortisol

To grasp the meaning of well-being at a physiological level, the reader has to have a good understanding of stress, chronic stress, how stress is triggered, and the short-term and long-term consequences of stress in relation to hedonic well-being.

Stress Stress is a state of physiological arousal involving the endocrine system, mostly in the form of adrenalin and cortisol. Specifically, the endocrine response during stress involves two parallel responses: the adrenocortical response (involving the sympathetic nervous system) and the adrenomedullary response (involving the hypothalamus and pituitary) (Lovallo, 2016, pp. 57–62).

The stress response system serves to deal with organismic threats and eventually to restore homeostasis—return the body to a normal state (Lovallo, 2016). Stress is customarily viewed as a state of physiological disharmony (imbalance) triggered by a stressor, psychological or physical threat. A psychological threat is usually a perceived adverse circumstance from the external environment (e.g., a physical attack by a predator) or it can originate internally as an infection or some other disease symptom (McEwen & Wingfield, 2003) or perhaps even an imaginary threat—a threat created by one's own imagination.

The Anatomy of Stress The stress response system involves two subsystems: the autonomic nervous system (ANS) and the peripheral autonomic system (PNS). The ANS subsystem serves is to slow down functions of all internal organs to conserve and redirect energy to deal with the stress. The ANS is triggered by signals from the limbic and other higher brain regions in the form of negative affect (fear, anger, panic, anxiety, etc.), which in turn triggers a stress response (in the form of pupil dilation, paleness, tachycardia, etc.). The PNS involves two processes: sympathetic and parasympathetic. These systems have conflicting goals—the sympathetic system prepares the body for the fight-or-flight response, whereas the parasympathetic system brings back the body to normal functioning after the source of stress is treated. As such, the body restores homeostasis (e.g., Chrousos & Gold, 1992).

Short-Term Versus Long-Term Consequences of Stress A feature of homeostasis involves "heterostasis" (Selye, 1956). Heterostasis refers to the mobilization of defensive mechanisms that stimulate the physiologic adaptive mechanisms to counter internal or environmental threats. When the threat has not been removed or neutralized, maintaining homeostasis becomes a source of ongoing wear-and-tear on the system. This is what is commonly referred to as "allostasis" (e.g., Sterling & Eyer, 1988)—continuing force acting against homeostasis causing the individual to continually expend additional resources to maintain homeostasis but at a systemic cost on well-being. In other words, allostasis is deleterious to mental (and physical) health because ongoing threats reduce the individual's ability to cope psychologically (and physiologically) with new major threats.

The endocrine response during stress is regulated by *cortisol*. As such, homeostasis involves the regulatory action of cortisol, which is fundamental to normal functioning, daily activities, and survival in general. In contrast, allostasis involves repeatedly elevated and greatly prolonged high levels of cortisol (i.e., chronic stress), ultimately affecting mental well-being. This occurs through amygdala sensitization and loss of hippocampal volume, both associated with the formation and consolidation of long-term memory of adverse events (Lovallo, 2016, p. 132). Specifically, when the amygdala is exposed to chronic stress it becomes sensitized to aversive or threatening stimuli rendering the entire central nervous system highly reactive to fight-or-flight events. This *amygdala-sensitization effect* is associated with post-traumatic stress disorder (e.g., Bremner et al., 1995). In other words, stress-induced changes in cognition and memory exert a long-term effect on stress reactivity and well-being (both physiological and psychological). Repeatedly elevated and greatly prolonged high levels of cortisol is also associated with *shrinkage of hippocampal volume* (e.g., Gilbertson et al., 2002). Patients with post-traumatic stress disorder have reduced hippocampal volume. The hippocampus is the primary site of negative feedback for cortisol regulation. Also, it is important to note that disease, frailty, and disability have a direct toll of the stress response in that individuals afflicted with disease, frailty, and/or disability are likely to experience allostasis—continuing force acting against homeostasis causing the individual to continually expend additional resources to maintain homeostasis but at a systemic cost on mental well-being (e.g., McEwen & Wingfield, 2003; Rockwood, Hogan, & MacKnight, 2000).

The Relationship Between Stress and Hedonic Well-Being Much research has demonstrated that positive emotions serve as stress buffers the deleterious effects of stress on the immune system (see literature review in Hostinar & Gunnar, 2013). For example, social stress, especially early in life, produces high levels of cortisol responses during social interactions and long-standing reductions in serotonin levels, underscoring the relationship between neurochemicals associated with positive and negative emotions (Spinelli et al., 2012). In a meta-analytic study, Pressman and Cohen (2005) found a negative relationship between dispositional positive affect and cortisol—the higher the dispositional positive affect the lower the cortisol. In sum, a good way to view the relationship between stress and hedonic well-being is to anchor our understanding on the concepts of homeostasis and allostasis. The stress response system is essentially a motivational system. Adverse environmental stimuli (such as threats) create homeostatic imbalance which motivates the individual to restore homeostasis. Removing the noxious stimuli reduces the flow of cortisol in the system and in many situations increases the flow of certain neurotransmitters in the brain's reward center, neurotransmitters such as dopamine and serotonin. Such outcome increases momentary hedonic well-being. Positive environmental stimuli (such as resources) also trigger homeostatic imbalance motivating the individual to take action to acquire the noted resources. Similarly, restoring homeostatic balance in this case increases the flow the positive neurotransmitters that activate the reward center in the brain, which in turn contributes to a momentary sense of well-being. In the long run, repeated and prolonged exposure to environmental threats produces an overflow of cortisol in the system, which in turn takes a toll on dispositional dimensions of well-being. And conversely, repeated and prolonged exposure to environmental resources produces an overflow of positive neurotransmitters in the system, which in turn contributes to the individuals' dispositional well-being.

Conclusion

In this chapter, I offered a definition of positive mental health at the physiological level. Individuals with high levels of well-being (specifically neurochemicals associated with rewards and stress) experience a preponderance of neurochemicals related to rewards (dopamine, serotonin, and oxytocin.) relative to negative neurochemicals related to stress (cortisol), at the physiological level. This definition of positive mental health at the physiological level is based on much of the research literature on the neurobiology of hedonic well-being and the stress response system.

The next chapter will focus on positive balance as viewed from an emotional level of analysis. I will focus on the concept of hedonic well-being (i.e., positive and negative affect) and show that positive and negative affect (well-being at the emotional level) is a phenomenon formed by the interplay of neurochemicals associated with rewards/stress and a process involving cognitive appraisal. A definition of positive balance at the emotional level is discussed with supportive evidence from three programs of research: positive and negative affect, the broaden-and-build theory of positive emotions, and flow theory.

References

Aderem, A. (2005). Systems biology: Its practice and challenges. *Cell, 121*(4), 511–513.

Advokat, C. D., Comaty, J. E., & Julien, R. M. (2014). *Julien's primer of drug action: A comprehensive guide to the actions, uses, and side effects of psychoactive drugs* (13th ed.). NY: Worth Publishers.

Austin, A., Jiga-Boy, G. M., Rea, S., Newstead, S. A., Roderick, S., Davis, N. J., et al. (2016). Prefrontal electrical stimulation in non-depressed reduces levels of reported negative effects from daily stressors. *Frontiers in Psychology, 7*(315).

Berns, G. S., McClure, S. M., Pagnoni, G., & Montague, P. R. (2001). Predictability modulates human brain response to reward. *Journal of Neuroscience, 21*, 2793–2798.

Brake, W. G., Zhang, T. Y., Diorio, J., Meaney, M. J., & Gratton, A. (2004). Influence of early postnatal rearing conditions on mesocorticolimbic dopamine and behavioural responses to psychostimulants and stressors in adult rats. *European Journal of Neuroscience, 19*, 1863–1874.

Bremner, J. D., Randall, P., Scott, T. M., Bronen, R. A., Seibyl, J. P., Southwick, S. M., et al. (1995). MRI-based measurement of hippocampal volume in patients with combat-related posttraumatic stress disorder. *American Journal of Psychiatry, 152*, 973–981.

Chrousos, G. P., & Gold, P. W. (1992). The concepts of stress and stress system disorders: Overview of physical and behavioral homeostasis. *Journal of the American Medical Association, 267*, 1244–1252.

Coccaro, R. M., & Kavoussi, R. J. (1997). Fluoxetine and impulsive aggressive behaviour in personality-disordered subjects. *Archives of General Psychiatry, 54*, 1081–1088.

Crommelinck, M., Feltz, B., & Goujon, P. (Eds.). (2006). *Self-organization and emergence in life sciences*. Heidelberg: Springer.

Dyer, K. R., & Cruickshank, C. C. (2005). Depression and other psychological health problems among methamphetamine dependent patients in treatment: Implications for assessment and treatment outcome. *Australian Psychologist, 40*, 96–108.

Elkins, D. N. (2016). *The human elements of psychotherapy: A nonmedical model of emotional healing*. Washington, DC: American Psychological Association.

Gianoulakis, C. (2001). Influence of the endogenous opioid system on high alcohol consumption and genetic predisposition to alcoholism. *Journal of Psychiatry & Neuroscience, 26*(4), 304–318.

Gilbertson, M. W., Shenton, M. E., Ciszewski, A., Kasai, K., Lasko, N. B., Orr, S. P., et al. (2002). Smaller hippocampal volume predicts pathologic vulnerability to psychological trauma. *Nature Neuroscience, 5*, 1242–1247.

Gratz, K. L., & Gunderson, J. G. (2006). Preliminary data on an acceptance-based emotion regulation group intervention for deliberate self-harm among women with borderline personality disorder. *Behavior Therapy, 37*, 25–35.

Hostinar, C. E., & Gunnar, M. R. (2013). Future directions in the study of social relationships as regulators of the HPA axis across development. *Journal of Clinical Child and Adolescent Psychology, 42*, 564–575.

Huppert, F. A. (2009). Psychological well-being: Evidence regarding its causes and consequences. *Applied Psychology: Health and Well-Being, 1*, 137–164.

Jackson, P. A., Sirgy, M. J., & Medley, G. D. (2018). The neurobiology of well-being. In N. R. Silton (Ed.), *Scientific concepts behind happiness, kindness and empathy in contemporary society* (pp. 135–155). Hershey, PA: IGI Global.

Jacobs, N., Delespaul, P., Derom, C., van Os, J., Myin-Germeys, I., & Nicolson, N. A. (2007). A momentary assessment study of the relationship between affective and adrenocortical stress responses in daily life. *Biological Psychology, 74*, 60–66.

Kalivas, P. W., & Volkow, N. D. (2005). The neural basis of addiction: A pathology of motivation and choice. *American Journal of Psychiatry, 162*, 1403–1413.

Kalivas, P. W., Peters, J., & Knackstedt, L. (2006). Animal models and brain circuits in drug addiction. *Molecular Interventions, 6*, 339–344.

Kasanetz, F., Deroche-Gamonet, V., Berson, N., Balado, E., Lafourcade, M., Manzoni, O., et al. (2010). Transition to addiction is associated with a persistent impairment in synaptic plasticity. *Science, 328*, 1709–1712.

Kendrick, K. M. (2004). The neurobiology of social bonds. *Neuroendocrinology, 16*, 1007–1008.

Kolb, B., & Whishaw, I. Q. (2014). *An introduction to brain and behaviour* (4th ed.). New York: Worth Publishers.

Kosfeld, M., Heinrichs, M., Zak, P. J., Fischbacher, U., & Fehr, E. (2005). Oxytocin increases trust in humans. *Nature, 435*, 673–676.

Looby, A., & Earleywine, M. (2007). The impact of methamphetamine use on subjective well-being in an internet survey: Preliminary findings. *Human Psychopharmacology, 22*, 167–172.

Lovallo, W. R. (2016). *Stress & health: Biological and psychological interactions*. Thousand Oaks, CA: Sage Publications.

Mathew, J., & Paulose, C. S. (2011). The healing power of well-being. *Acta Neuropsychiatrica, 23*, 145–155.

McEwen, B. S., & Wingfield, J. C. (2003). The concept of allostasis in biology and biomedicine. *Hormones and Behavior, 43*, 2–15.

McKim, W. A., & Hancock, S. (2013). *Drugs and behavior* (7th ed.). Upper Saddle River, NJ: Pearson Prentice Hall.

McRae-Clark, A. L., Baker, N. L., Maria, M. M., & Brady, K. T. (2013). Effect of oxytocin on craving and stress response in marijuana-dependent individuals: A pilot study. *Psychopharmacology, 228*, 623–631.

Nestler, E. (2005). Is there a common molecular pathway for addiction? *Nature Neuroscience, 8*, 1445–1449.

Olds, J., & Milner, P. (1954). Positive reinforcement produced by electrical stimulation of septal area and other regions of the brain. *Journal of Comparative and Physiological Psychology, 47*, 419–427.

Panksepp, J. (2005). Affective consciousness: Core emotional feelings in animals and humans. *Consciousness and Cognition, 14*, 30–80.

Patil, S., Sen, S., Bral, M., Reddy, S., Bradley, K. K., Cornett, E. M., et al. (2016). The role of acupuncture in pain management. *Current Pain and Headache Reports, 20*, 22–30.

Pedersen, C. A., Smedley, K. L., Leserman, J., Jarskog, L. F., Rau, S. W., Kampov-Polevoi, A., et al. (2013). Intranasal oxytocin blocks alcohol withdrawal in human subjects. *Alcohol Clinical and Experimental Research, 37*, 484–489.

Peirson, A. R., & Heuchert, J. W. (2000). Correlations for serotonin levels and measures of mood in a nonclinical sample. *Psychological Reports, 87*, 707–716.

Petrocchi, N., Piccirillo, G., Fiorucci, C., Moscucci, F., Iorio, C., Mastropietri, F., et al. (2017). Transcranial direct current stimulation enhances soothing positive affect and vagal tone. *Neuropsychologia, 96*, 256–261.

Polk, D. E., Skoner, D. P., Kirschbaum, C., Cohen, S., & Doyle, W. J. (2005). State and trait affect as predictors of salivary cortisol in healthy adults. *Psychoneuroendocrinology, 30*, 261–272.

Pressman, S. D., & Cohen, S. (2005). Does positive affect influence health? *Psychological Bulletin, 131*, 925–971.

Pruessner, J. C., Hellhammer, D. H., & Kirschbaum, C. (1999). Low self-esteem induced failure and the adrenocortical stress response. *Personality and Individual Differences, 27*, 477–489.

Rickard, N. S., & Vella-Brodrick, D. A. (2014). Changes in well-being: Complementing a psychosocial approach with neurobiological insights. *Social Indicators Research, 117*, 437–457.

Robinson, T. E., & Berridge, K. C. (1993). The neural basis of drug craving: An incentive-sensitization theory of addiction. *Brain Research Reviews, 18*, 247–291.

Robinson, T. E., & Berridge, K. C. (2001). Incentive-sensitization and addiction. *Addiction, 96*, 103–114.

Robinson, T. E., & Berridge, K. C. (2003). Addiction. *Annual Review of Psychology, 54*, 25–53.

Rockwood, K., Hogan, D. B., & MacKnight, C. (2000). Conceptualisation and measurement of frailty in elderly people. *Drugs & Aging, 17*, 295–302.

Schultz, W. (2002). Getting formal with dopamine and reward. *Neuron, 36*, 241–263.

Schultz, W. (2010). Dopamine signals for reward value and risk: Basic and recent data. *Behavioral and Brain Functions, 6*, 24.

Selye, H. (1956). *The stress of life*. New York: McGraw-Hill.

Siever, D. (2015). Stimulation technologies: "New" trends in "old" techniques. *Biofeedback, 43*, 180–192.

Silton, N. R., Flannelly, L. T., Flannelly, K. J., & Galek, K. (2011). Toward a theory of holistic needs and the brain. *Holistic Nursing Practice, 25*, 258–265.

Smyth, J., Ockenfels, M. C., Porter, L., Kirschbaum, C., Hellhammer, D. H., & Stone, A. A. (1998). Stressors and mood measured on a momentary basis are associated with salivary cortisol secretion. *Psychoneuroendocrinology, 23*, 353–370.

Solé, R. V., Ferrer-Cancho, R., Montoya, J. M., & Valverde, S. (2002). Selection, tinkering, and emergence in complex networks. *Complexity, 8*(1), 20–33.

Spanagel, D. V., & Weiss, F. (1999). The dopamine hypothesis of reward: Past and current status. *Trends in Neuroscience, 22*, 521–527.

Spinelli, S., Schwandt, M. L., Lindell, S. G., Heilig, M., Suomi, S. J., Higley, J. D., et al. (2012). The serotonin transporter gene linked polymorphic region is associated with the behavioral response to repeated stress exposure in infant rhesus macaques. *Developmental and Psychopathology, 24*, 157–165.

Sterling, P., & Eyer, J. (1988). Allostasis: A new paradigm to explain arousal pathology. In S. Fisher & J. Reason (Eds.), *Handbook of life stress, cognition, and health* (pp. 629–649). New York, NY: Wiley.

Stagg, C. J., Best, J. G., Stephenson, M. C., O'Shea, J., Wylezinska, M., Kincses, Z. T., et al. (2009). Polarity-sensitive modulation of cortical neurotransmitters by transcranial stimulation. *The Journal of Neuroscience, 29*, 5202–5206.

Volkow, N. D., Wang, G.-J., Ma, Y., Fowler, J. S., Wong, C., Ding, Y.-S., et al. (2005). Activation of orbital and medial prefrontal cortex by methylphenidate in cocaine-addicted subjects but not in controls: Relevance to addiction. *Journal of Neuroscience, 25*, 3932–3939.

Volkow, N. D., Wang, G.-J., Telang, F., Fowler, J. S., Alexoff, D., Logan, J., et al. (2014). Decreased dopamine brain reactivity in marijuana abusers is associated with negative emotionality and addiction severity. *Proceedings of the National Academy of Sciences*, E3149–E3156.

Wang, G.-J., Volkow, N. D., Fowler, J. S., Cervany, P., Hitzemann, R. J., Pappas, N. R., et al. (1999). Regional brain metabolic activation during craving elicited by recall of previous drug experiences. *Life Science, 64*, 775–784.

Wenk, G. L. (2009). *Your brain on food: How chemicals control your thoughts and feelings*. New York: Oxford University Press.

Wilder, J. (1958). Modern psychophysiology and the law of initial value. *American Journal of Psychotherapy, 12*, 199–221.

Williams, E., Stewart-Knox, B., Helander, A., McConville, C., Bradbury, I., & Rowland, I. (2006). Associations between whole-blood serotonin and subjective mood in healthy male volunteers. *Biological Psychology, 71*, 171–174.

Wise, R. A. (1996). Addictive drugs and brain stimulation reward. *Annual Review of Neuroscience, 19*, 319–340.

Zelkowitz, P., Gold, I., Feeley, N., Hayton, B., Carter, C. S., Tulandi, T., et al. (2014). Psychosocial stress moderates the relationships between oxytocin, perinatal depression, and maternal behavior. *Hormones and Behavior, 66*, 351–360.

Chapter 3
Positive Balance at the Emotional Level: Hedonic Well-Being

Introduction

> Positivity opens us. The first core truth about positive emotions is that they open our hearts and our minds, making us more receptive and more creative.—Barbara Fredrickson (https://www.azquotes.com/author/26164-Barbara_Fredrickson)

To remind the reader, in Chap. 1, I offered a definition of positive mental health from an emotional perspective. This definition reflects my view of positive balance. Here is the definition again. Individuals who have positive mental health at the emotional level tend to experience *a preponderance of positive emotions (pleasure, happiness, joy, contentment, vitality, etc.) relative to negative emotions (anger, sadness, jealousy, envy, hatred, grief, isolation, worthlessness, etc.).*

In this chapter, I discuss research that supports this definition of positive mental health at the emotional level. I refer to three research programs, namely positive and negative affect, the broaden-and-build theory and flow. I briefly discussed these two programs of research in Chap. 1, but I delve in greater detail in this chapter. I will then discuss the concept of emergence that links well-being at the physiological level (neurochemicals associated with the reward center and the stress response system) with well-being at the emotional level (hedonic well-being or positive and negative affect). I conclude by making the following assertion: Positive neurochemicals (dopamine, serotonin, and oxytocin) at the physiological level mediated by a process of cognitive appraisal (positive frame) result into positive affect (happiness, joy, contentment, etc.) at the emotional level; and conversely, negative neurochemicals (cortisol) mediated by a process of cognitive appraisal (negative frame) result into negative affect (anger, sadness, jealousy, envy, depression, etc. See the shaded row in Table 3.1.

© Springer Nature Switzerland AG 2020
M. J. Sirgy, *Positive Balance*, Social Indicators Research Series 80,
https://doi.org/10.1007/978-3-030-40289-1_3

Table 3.1 Positive mental health defined at various hierarchical levels as positive balance with emergence and focus on the emotional level

Level of analysis	Positive balance as positive mental health	Programs of research	Emergence
Positive mental health defined at a physiological level = **positive and negative neurotransmitters**	Individuals experiencing a preponderance of neurochemicals related to positive emotions (dopamine, serotonin, oxytocin) relative to neurochemicals related to negative emotions (cortisol)	Stress response system); neurobiology of happiness)	
Positive mental health defined at an emotional level = **positive/negative affect or hedonic well-being (positive/negative neurotransmitters + cognitive appraisals)**	Individuals experiencing a preponderance of positive emotions (happiness, joy, serenity, contentment, etc.) relative to negative emotions (anger, sadness, jealousy, envy, depression, etc.)	Positive versus negative affect; broaden and build theory; flow	Positive neurochemicals (dopamine, serotonin, and oxytocin) at the physiological level mediated by a process of cognitive appraisal (positive frame) result into positive affect (happiness, joy, contentment, etc.) at the emotional level; and conversely, negative neurochemicals (cortisol) mediated by a process of cognitive appraisal (negative frame) result into negative affect (anger, sadness, jealousy, envy, depression, etc.)
Positive mental health defined at a cognitive level = **domain satisfaction (positive/negative affect + domain segmentation)**	Individuals experiencing a preponderance of domain satisfaction (satisfaction in salient and multiple life domains such as family life, work life, social life, etc.) relative to dissatisfaction in other life domains	Principle of satisfaction limits; principle of the full spectrum of human developmental needs; principle of diminishing satisfaction	Positive affect (happiness, joy, contentment, etc.) at the emotional level mediated by a process of domain segmentation result into domain satisfaction (satisfied with work life, social life, family life, etc.); and conversely, negative affect (anger, sadness, jealousy, envy, depression, etc.) mediated by a process of domain segmentation result into domain dissatisfaction (dissatisfied with work life, social life, family life, etc.)
Positive mental health defined at a meta-cognitive level = **life satisfaction (domain satisfaction + bottom-up process)**	Individuals experiencing a preponderance of positive evaluations about one's life using certain standards of comparison (satisfaction with one's life compared to one's past life, the life of family members, the life of associates at work, the life of others in the same social circles, etc.) relative to negative evaluations about one's life using similar or other standards of comparison	Multiple discrepancies theory; congruity life satisfaction; temporal life satisfaction; social comparison; frequency of positive affect; homeostatically protected mood	Domain satisfaction (satisfied with work life, social life, family life, etc.) at the cognitive level mediated by a bottom-up process at the meta-cognitive level result in life satisfaction; and conversely. domain dissatisfaction (dissatisfied with work life, social life, family life, etc.) mediated by a bottom-up process result in life dissatisfaction

(continued)

Table 3.1 (continued)

Positive mental health defined at a developmental level = **eudaimonia (life satisfaction + personal growth)**	Individuals experiencing a preponderance of positive psychological traits (self-acceptance, personal growth, purpose in life, environmental mastery, autonomy, positive relations with others, etc.) relative to negative psychological traits (pessimism, hopelessness, depressive disorder, neuroticism, impulsiveness, etc.)	Hedonic versus eudaimonic happiness; virtue ethics and character strengths; self-determination theory; personal expressiveness; psychological well-being; purpose and meaning in life; flourishing; orientations to happiness; resilience; and satisfaction of the full spectrum of human needs	Life satisfaction at the meta-cognitive level mediated by a process involving high personal growth result in high levels of eudaimonia at the developmental level; and conversely, life dissatisfaction mediated by a process involving low personal growth result into low levels of eudaimonia
Positive mental health defined at a social-ecological level = **socio-eudaimonia (eudaimonia + social & moral development)**	Individuals experiencing a preponderance of social resources (social acceptance, social actualization, social contribution, social integration, social harmony, social belonginess, social attachment, familial attachment, etc.) relative to social constraints (social alienation, social discord, social exclusion, ostracism, etc.)	Social well-being, social harmony need to belong, attachment theory; social exclusion and ostracism	High levels of eudaimonia at the developmental level mediated by a process involving high social and moral development result into high levels of socio-eudaimonia at the social-ecological level; and conversely, low levels of eudaimonia mediated by a process involving low social and moral development result into low levels of socio-eudaimonia

Programs of Research Supporting the Definition of Positive Balance

In the sections below I will discuss three programs of research supporting the definition of positive mental health at the emotional level. These are positive versus negative affect, broaden and build theory, and flow.

Positive and Negative Affect

Some well-being scientists (e.g., Diener, Smith, & Fujita, 1995) treat well-being as a psychological state involving a preponderance of positive affect (e.g., joy, contentment, pleasure) over negative (e.g., sadness, depression, anxiety, anger). To better understand this conception of well-being, let us review the research on the conceptualization and measurement of positive and negative affect. The concept of well-being is captured by measuring two types of affect, positive and negative, and then summing up the scores to derive an index of well-being (e.g., Bradburn, 1969;

Table 3.2 A scale measuring positive and negative affect

Please think about what you have been doing and experiencing during the past 4 weeks. The report how much you experienced each of the following feelings, using the scale below. For each item, select a number from 1 to 5, and indicate that number on your response sheet
1 = very rarely or never
2 = rarely
3 = sometimes
4 = often
5 = very often or always
• Positive
• Negative
• Good
• Bad
• Pleasant
• Unpleasant
• Happy
• Sad
• Afraid
• Joyful
• Angry
• Contented
Scoring: The measure can be used to derive an overall affect balance score but can also be divided into positive and negative feeling scales
Positive feelings (SPANE-P): Add the scores varying from 1 to 5, for the six items: positive, good, pleasant, happy, joyful, and contented. The score can vary from 6 (lowest possible) to 30 (highest possible)
Negative feelings (SPANE-N): Add the scores varying from 1 to 5, for the six items: negative, bad, unpleasant, sad, afraid, and angry. The score can vary from 6 (lowest possible) to 30 (highest possible)
Affect balance (SPANE-B): The negative feelings score is subtracted from the positive feelings score, and the resultant difference score can vary from −24 (unhappiness possible) to 24 (happiest possible)

Source: Adapted from Diener et al. (2010)

Chamberlain, 1988; Diener, Smith, & Fujita, 1995; Headey, Kelley, & Wearing, 1993; Kim & Mueller, 2001; Lucas, Diener, & Suh, 1996; Watson, Clark, & Tellegen, 1988). That is, a person who has a high level of well-being is one who has a preponderance of positive affect (such as joy, contentment, or pleasure) over negative affect (such as sadness, depression, anxiety, or anger).

See example of a positive/negative affect measure in Table 3.2. Another measure commonly used to capture positive and negative affect is the *Intensity and Time Affect Scale* (ITAS; Diener et al., 1995). The ITAS is a 24-item measure capturing how frequently respondents have experienced different positive (e.g., joy, affection) and negative (e.g., anger, fear) emotions. Subjects respond to a 7-point rating scale in which "1" denotes "never experience" and "7" representing "always experience."

Table 3.3 Measuring hedonic sensations of momentary pleasures

Ecological momentary assessment
Participants are given a sampling diary and are instructed to rate their current feelings on a series of affect adjectives (happy, tired, stressed, frustrated, and angry) on 5-point scales (1 = not at all, and 5 = very much) at 6 time points: At the office, at bedtime, 30 min after waking the next morning, noon, and at 3 pm
Day reconstruction method
A diary is completed online at the end of each 24 h period. Participants are asked to recall the monitoring period as a continuous series of episodes (e.g., similar to episodes of a television show). Each episode is defined in terms of time of onset and duration, location, social situation, and activity. After the complete 24 h are reconstructed, participants rate their feelings related to each episode on a series of affective states (happy, tired, worry, feeling hassled, angry, and frustrated) on 7-point scales (0 = not at all and 6 = very much)

Source: Adapted from Dockray and Steptoe (2010)

Daniel Kahneman, a Nobel Laureate and a leading scholar in the psychology of well-being research, has conceptualized happiness as sensations associated with real-time feelings of happiness (Kahneman, 1999). He calls it "objective happiness." To measure this concept, he employs an *experiential sampling method*. Subjects are contacted at set time intervals during the day and asked to report their positive and negative feelings they experience at the time of the contact (or during the last hour or so). See two example measures in Table 3.3.

The concepts of positive and negative affect capture what some well-being researchers call *emotional well-being* at a macro level. Şimşek (2011) has argued that the traditional measures capturing happiness in terms of positive and negative affect (e.g., the PANAS measure; Watson et al., 1988) do not refer to "life" as object of evaluation. Therefore, the author developed a measure combining positive and negative affect with references to life at large. The exact measure is shown in Table 3.4.

The reader should note that there is much evidence indicating that measures of positive and negative affect are highly correlated to measures of domain satisfaction and life satisfaction (e.g., Diener, Emmons, Larsen, & Griffin, 1985; Emmons & Diener, 1985; Tsou & Liu, 2001). This stream of research suggests that individuals experiencing a preponderance of positive over negative affect are likely to experience greater satisfaction in various life domains as well as life overall. As such, this research provides support to the positive balance view of positive mental health at the emotional level—individuals experiencing a preponderance of positive emotions (happiness, joy, serenity, contentment, etc.) relative to negative emotions (anger, sadness, jealousy, envy, depression, etc.).

Table 3.4 An emotional well-being scale

Positive emotional well-being
• Life gives me pleasure
• Life excites me
• I feel at peace with life
• I am content with life
• I appreciate the life I lead
• I completely accept life as it is
Negative emotional well-being
• I feel pain about my life
• I feel upset about my life
• The life I lead gets me down
• The life I lead frightens me
• I worry about the life I lead
• The life I lead saddens me
• I feel I'm wasting my life
Response scale: 5-point Likert scale varying from "1 = strong disagree" to "5 = strongly agree"

Source: Adapted from Şimşek (2011), p. 425)

Broaden-and-Build Theory of Positive Emotions

The *broaden-and-build theory of positive emotions* (e.g., Fredrickson, 2001, 2004; Fredrickson & Joiner, 2002) asserts that positive emotions serve to broaden an individuals' momentary thought-action repertoire. Positive emotions induce playfulness, exploratory behavior, savoring experiences, creativity, close connections and bonding with others, engagement in approach behaviors, among other positive behavioral outcomes. In contrast, negative emotions (associated with the visceral fight-or-flight response) prompt the individual to contract cognitively, socially, and engage in avoidance behaviors. The broadening of the thought-action repertoire through positive emotions allows the individual to build personal resources—physical resources, intellectual resources, social resources, psychological resources, etc. These resources serve the individual in many ways to enhance functioning. Furthermore, these resources serve as reserves that can be drawn on to help deal with adversity. As such, these resources enhance personal resilience.

For example, in an organizational context, Wright (2010) uses the *broaden-and-build theory* to explain the effects of employee well-being (and psychological well-being) on a host of employee cognitive/affective/conative responses as well as other organizational outcomes. Positive emotions (i.e., positivity) serve to broaden the employee's momentary thought-action repertoires by expanding an array of thoughts and actions in the workplace. In contrast, negative emotions (i.e., negativity) diminish the same mechanisms and outcomes. Employees experiencing a high level of positivity than negativity tend to be more creative, outgoing, and sociable than those experiencing negativity. Positive employees tend to remember favorable events better and are less likely to interpret ambiguous events as threatening compared to negative employees. Positivity also helps employees build personal resources of all kinds—physical, emotional, intellectual, and social resources. These personal resources help them thrive in the workplace in many ways. Thus, positivity can account for higher job performance, job involvement and effort, organizational commitment, work attendance, and prosocial and organizational citizenship behaviors. By the same token, positivity also accounts for lower levels of intention to quit, decisions to retire, employee turnover, and workplace incivility.

There is also evidence to suggest that it is not only positive emotions that produce positive behavioral outcomes but the preponderance of positive affect over negative affect (Fredrickson, 2009, 2013). People who "flourish" (those who are psychologically healthy) experience at least three times as many positive emotions as they do negative emotions. In contrast, the ratio is two-to-one for "nonflourishers."

But then the question is whether positive emotions contribute to positive mental health in a linear fashion. Research has addressed this question, and the answer is a resounding no. Too much positivity is not necessarily good for positive mental health [see discussion of this research question and evidence in Forgas (2014) and Fredrickson and Joiner (2002)]. The relationship looks more like an inverted-U. Too much positive emotions do not contribute to high levels mental well-being. Fredrickson (2013) argues that increasing positivity contributes to creativity, job performance, health, and other outcomes up to a certain level. After moderate levels of positive emotions, these behavioral outcomes diminish significantly. Some degree of negative emotions seems necessary to motivate people to take corrective action. Corrective action leads to positive behavioral outcomes (Catalino, Algoe, & Fredrickson, 2011; Fredrickson, 2013). This evidence points to the assertion that positive mental health reflects a preponderance of positive over negative emotions. That is, negative emotions must be part of this optimal state but significantly in lesser amount than positive emotions.

Flow

Besides the research on the broaden-and-build theory, much of the research on *flow* reflects the notion that well-being is associated with both positive and negative emotions (e.g., Csikszentmihalyi & LeFevre, 1989). Specifically, certain activities that are challenging and matching one's level of skills induce much positive emotions (positive emotions related to achievement, mastery, and efficacy) juxtaposed with negative emotions (frustration related to task difficulty, pain in the exertion of physical and mental effort, and perseverance in light of failure). Engaging in activities that produce flow contributes significantly to subjective well-being. Note that flow theory emphasizes the notion that the flow experience necessitates elements that call for negative affect (i.e., physical exertion, effort, and learning from failure experiences).

Flow theory asserts that work activities are pleasurable when the challenge is matched with the individual's skill level (Csikszentmihalyi, 1975). When an individual engages in an activity that is either too easy or too difficult, he or she is not likely to experience flow—a state of total absorption with the work activity. Csikszentmihalyi has argued repeatedly that a happy life is not an excellent life. To lead an excellent life is to engage in activities that help us grow and fulfill our potential (Csikszentmihalyi, 1975, 1982, 1990, 1997). In his book *Finding Flow*, he states:

> The quality of life does not depend on happiness alone, but also on what one does to be happy. If one fails to develop goals that give meaning to one's existence, if one does not use the mind to its fullest, then good feelings fulfill just a fraction of the potential we possess. A person who achieves contentment by withdrawing from the world "to cultivate his own garden," like Voltaire's *Candide*, cannot be said to lead an excellent life. Without dreams, without risks, only a trivial semblance of living can be achieved (Csikszentmihalyi, 1997, p. 22).

The research on flow and the quotation above underscores the notion that positive mental health at the emotional level involves both positive and negative affect. Engaging in activities that produce a sense of well-being (i.e., flow) typically involves a certain degree of displeasure (i.e., negative affect). As the saying goes, "no pain no gain." As such, the research provides support to the positive balance view of positive mental health at the emotional level—individuals experiencing a preponderance of positive emotions (happiness, joy, serenity, contentment, etc.) relative to negative emotions (anger, sadness, jealousy, envy, depression, etc.).

Emergence

As briefly mentioned in the opening part of the chapter, the research related to neurobiology of happiness and the stress response system leads us to a clear conclusion. This conclusion is captured by the following theoretical proposition: *Positive neurochemicals (dopamine, serotonin, and oxytocin) at the physiological level mediated by a process of cognitive appraisal (positive frame) result into positive affect (happiness, joy, contentment, etc.) at the emotional level; and conversely, negative neurochemicals (cortisol) mediated by a process of cognitive appraisal (negative frame) result into negative affect (anger, sadness, jealousy, envy, depression, etc.).*

Hedonic well-being is a subjective well-being concept that is best understood in the context of the hierarchy of concepts of well-being, specifically at the emotional level of the hierarchy. Hedonic well-being has been the focus of this chapter. As such, the reader should appreciate much of the discussion in this chapter by gaining a mental grasp of the link between well-being at the physiological level (neurochemicals associated with the reward center in the brain and the stress response system) and well-being at the emotional level (hedonic well-being or positive and negative affect). This link can be viewed in terms of emergence. As mentioned in Chap. 1, emergence is a concept well-entrenched in systems science, especially in biology and the life sciences. Specifically, emergence refers to higher-level systems

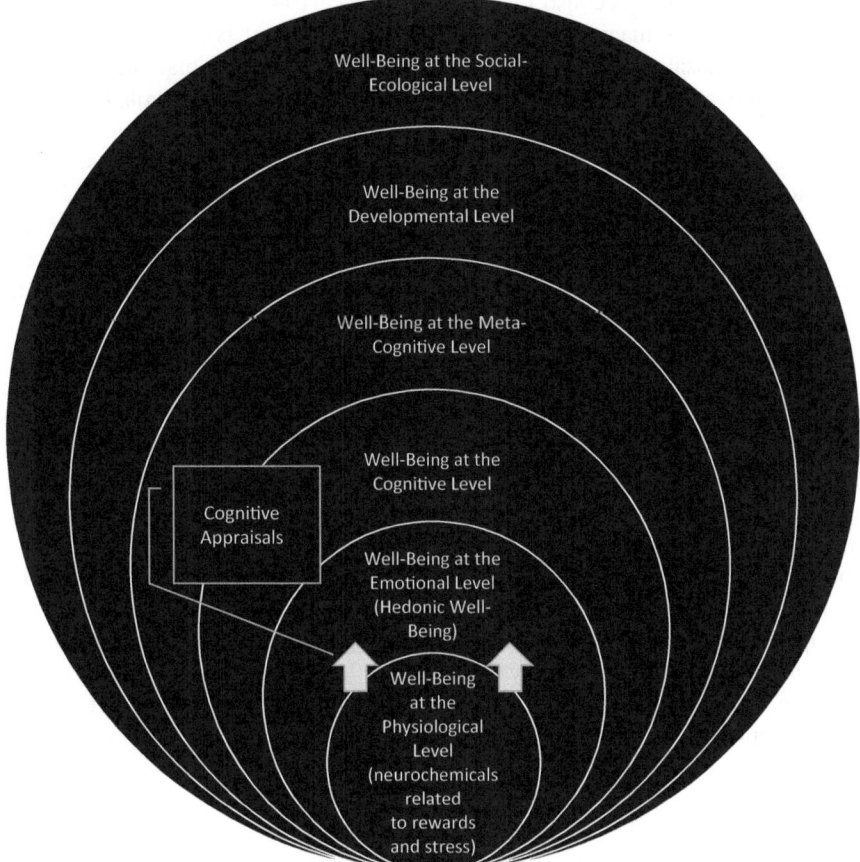

Fig. 3.1 Emergence: well-being at the emotional level (positive/negative affect) influenced by well-being at the physiological level (neurochemicals related to rewards and stress) mediated by a process of cognitive appraisal

"emerge" from lower-level systems. In other words, complex systems have "emergent properties" that are not inherent in their individual parts and cannot be understood even with full understanding of the parts alone. See Fig. 3.1.

So how does well-being at the physiological level (positive and negative neurochemicals) contribute to the formation and maintenance of well-being at the emotional level (positive and negative affect)? This occurs through a process of cognitive appraisal. That is, positive and negative affect (or hedonic well-being), commonly treated as the key concept of well-being at the emotional level, is an emergent property of positive and negative neurochemicals in the brain mediated by cognitive appraisals (Siemer, Mauss, & Gross, 2007). Much research has demonstrated that emotions are the direct result of cognitive appraisals of surges of neurochemicals in the brain. Consider the seminal work of Lazarus and his colleagues related to coping

(Lazarus, 1966, 1999; see also Lazarus & Folkman, 1984). Their research demonstrated that stress, as manifested in terms of surges of cortisol, is experienced through cognitive appraisal of one's available resources to deal with situational demands. Research has also demonstrated that stressors appraised as uncontrollable, novel, challenging, or threatening trigger a stress response. Moreover, specific cognitive appraisals produce specific emotional responses. These emotional responses, in turn, serve to mediate the effect of stressful events on the excretion of cortisol.

A meta-analysis of studies involving stress, cortisol, and cognitive appraisals (Denson, Spanovic, & Miller, 2009) was able to demonstrate that specific emotional responses associated with specific types of environmental demands influence cortisol in a manner that is adaptive to the survival of the human species. This research suggests that coping strategies that alter appraisals and emotional responses may improve long-term health outcomes, particularly in relation to stressors that are acute or imminent, threaten one's social status, or require extended effort. Stressors that are acute or imminent tend to be associated with cognitive appraisals and emotions such as surprise, anticipation, worry, disgust, and threat. Stressors that reflect threat to one's social status are associated with appraisals and emotions such as submissiveness, fearing loss of social approval, threat, ruination, and self-conscious emotions. Stressors that signal requirement of extended effort are associated with appraisals and emotions such as challenge, threat, intensity, novelty, surprise, and anticipation. With respect to positive emotions, much research has shown that pleasantness (e.g., Smith & Ellsworth, 1985) reflect an appraisal that the event or outcome is congruent or incongruent with the individual's wants or desires. If the event is appraised as congruent, then positive emotions such as joy and pride may be experienced.

Conclusion

I offered a definition of positive mental health at the emotional level. To reiterate, the definition is as follows: Individuals with high levels of well-being experience a preponderance of positive emotions (happiness, joy, elation, contentment, serenity, etc.) relative to negative emotions (anger, hate, disgust, fear, jealousy, envy, etc.). This definition of positive mental health at the emotional level is based on much of the research related to three programs of research in well-being, namely the measurement of positive and negative affect, the broaden-and-build theory of positive emotions, and flow theory.

I also explained how well-being at the physiological level (positive and negative neurochemical) influence the formation of well-being at the emotional level (hedonic well-being). I argued that positive neurochemicals (dopamine, serotonin, and oxytocin) at the physiological level mediated by a process of cognitive appraisal (positive frame) result into positive affect (happiness, joy, contentment, etc.) at the emotional level; and conversely, negative neurochemicals (cortisol) mediated by a process of cognitive appraisal (negative frame) result into negative affect (anger, sadness, jealousy, envy, depression, etc.

The next chapter focuses on positive balance as viewed from a cognitive level of analysis. I focus on the concept of domain satisfaction and show that domain satisfaction (well-being at the cognitive level) is a phenomenon formed by the interplay of positive/negative affect involving a process of domain segmentation. A definition of positive balance at the cognitive level will be discussed with supportive evidence based on three balance principles: the principle of satisfaction limits, the principle of the full spectrum of human developmental needs, and the principle of diminishing satisfaction.

References

Bradburn, N. M. (1969). *The structure of psychological well-being*. Chicago: Aldine.

Catalino, L. I., Algoe, S. B., & Fredrickson, B. L. (2011). Prioritizing positivity: An effective approach to pursuing happiness? *Emotion, 14*, 1155–1161.

Chamberlain, K. (1988). On the structure of subjective well-being. *Social Indicators Research, 20*, 581–604.

Csikszentmihalyi, M. (1975). *Beyond boredom and anxiety*. San Francisco: Jossey-Bass.

Csikszentmihalyi, M. (1982). Towards a psychology of optimal experience. In L. Wheeler (Ed.), *Review of personality and social psychology* (Vol. 2). Beverly Hills, CA: Sage.

Csikszentmihalyi, M. (1990). *Flow: The psychology of optimal experience*. New York: Harper Perennial.

Csikszentmihalyi, M. (1997). *Finding flow: The psychology of engagement with everyday life*. New York: Basic Books.

Csikszentmihalyi, M., & LeFevre, J. (1989). Optimal experience in work and leisure. *Journal of Personality and Social Psychology, 56*, 815–822.

Denson, T. F., Spanovic, M., & Miller, N. (2009). Cognitive appraisals and emotions predict cortisol and immune responses: A meta-analysis of acute laboratory social stressors and emotion inductions. *Psychological Bulletin, 135*, 823–853.

Diener, E., Emmons, R. A., Larsen, R. J., & Griffin, S. (1985). The satisfaction with life scale. *Journal of Personality Assessment, 49*, 71–75.

Diener, E., Smith, H., & Fujita, F. (1995). The personality structure of affect. *Journal of Personality and Social Psychology, 69*, 130–141.

Diener, E., Wirtz, D., Tov, W., Kim-Prieto, C., Choi, D., Oishi, S., et al. (2010). New well-being measures: Short scales to assess flourishing and positive and negative feelings. *Social Indicators Research, 97*, 143–156.

Dockray, S., & Steptoe, A. (2010). Positive affect and psychobiological processes. *Neuroscience & Behavioral Review, 35*, 129–148.

Emmons, R. A., & Diener, E. (1985). Factors predicting satisfaction judgments: A comparative examination. *Social Indicators Research, 16*(2), 157–167.

Forgas, J. P. (2014). On the downside of feeling good: Evidence for the motivational, cognitive, and behavioral disadvantages of positive affect. In J. Gruber & J. T. Moskowitz (Eds.), *Positive emotion: Integrating the light sides and the dark sides* (pp. 301–322). New York: Oxford University Press.

Fredrickson, B. L. (2001). The role of positive emotions in positive psychology: The broaden-and-build theory of positive emotions. *American Psychologist, 56*, 218–222.

Fredrickson, B. L. (2004). The broaden-and-build theory of positive emotions. *Philosophical Transactions of the Royal Society B: Biological Sciences, 359*(1449), 1367–1377.

Fredrickson, B. L. (2009). *Positivity: Top-notch research reveals the 3-to-1 ratio that will change your life*. New York: Three Rivers Press.

Fredrickson, B. L. (2013). Updated thinking on positivity ratios. *American Psychologist, 68*, 814–822.

Fredrickson, B. L., & Joiner, T. (2002). Positive emotions trigger upward spirals toward emotional well-being. *Psychological Science, 13*, 172–175.

Headey, B., Kelley, J., & Wearing, A. (1993). Dimensions of mental health: Life satisfaction, positive affect, anxiety and depression. *Social Indicators Research, 29*, 63–82.

Kahneman, D. (1999). Objective happiness. In D. Kahneman, E. Diener, & N. Schwartz (Eds.), *Well-being: The foundations of hedonic psychology* (pp. 3–25). New York: Russell Sage Foundation.

Kim, K. A., & Mueller, D. J. (2001). To balance or not balance: Confirmatory factor analysis of the affect-balance scale. *Journal of Happiness Studies, 2*, 289–306.

Lazarus, R. S. (1966). *Psychological stress and the coping process*. New York: McGraw-Hill.

Lazarus, R. S. (1999). *Stress and emotion: A new synthesis*. New York: Springer.

Lazarus, R. S., & Folkman, S. (1984). *Stress, appraisal, and coping*. New York: Springer.

Lucas, R. E., Diener, E., & Suh, E. (1996). Discriminant validity of well-being measures. *Journal of Personality and Social Psychology, 71*, 616–628.

Siemer, M., Mauss, I., & Gross, J. J. (2007). Same situation—different emotions: How appraisals shape our emotions. *Emotion, 7*, 592–610.

Şimşek, Ö. F. (2011). An intentional model of emotional well-being: The development and initial validation of a measure of subjective well-being. *Journal of Happiness Studies, 12*(3), 421–442.

Smith, C. A., & Ellsworth, P. C. (1985). Patterns of cognitive appraisal in emotion. *Journal of Personality and Social Psychology, 48*, 813–838.

Tsou, M. W., & Liu, J. T. (2001). Happiness and domain satisfaction in Taiwan. *Journal of Happiness Studies, 2*(3), 269–288.

Watson, D., Clark, L. A., & Tellegen, A. (1988). Development and validation of brief measures of positive and negative affect: The PANAS scales. *Journal of Personality and Social Psychology, 54*, 1063–1070.

Wright, T. A. (2010). More than meets the eye: The role of employee well-being in organizational research. In P. A. Linlley, S. Harrington, & N. Garcea (Eds.), *Oxford handbook of positive psychology and work* (pp. 143–154). Oxford: Oxford University Press.

Chapter 4
Positive Balance at the Cognitive Level: Domain Satisfaction

Introduction

> Balance is not better time management, but better boundary management. Balance means making choices and enjoying those choices.—Betsy Jacobson (https://www. thebalancecareers.com/inspirational-quotes-about-work-life-balance-2062850)

Much research has been documented about concepts related to the balanced life in the literatures of organizational/industrial psychology and human resource management. These concepts include work-life balance, work-family balance, work-family interference, and work-family interface (see literature reviews of various concepts related to work-life balance by Allen, Herst, Bruck, & Sutton, 2000; Bulger & Fisher, 2012; Byron, 2005; Casper, Eby, Bordeaux, Lockwood, & Lambert, 2007; Danna & Griffin, 1999; Eby, Casper, Lockwood, Bordeaux, & Brinley, 2005, Eby, Maher, & Butts, 2010; Greenhaus & Allen, 2011; Kalliath & Brough, 2008; Kossek & Ozeki, 1998; Lee & Sirgy, 2017; McNall, Nicklin, & Masuda, 2010; Sirgy & Lee, 2016, 2018a; Sirgy, Reilly, Wu, & Efraty, 2008; Yasbek, 2004). In the literature of subjective well-being, only a few studies were found addressing life balance. For example, Diener, Ng, and Tov (2008) reported a study involving a representative sample of the world to assess people's affect balance (positive versus negative affect) on the previous day and the various activities they have engaged in. The study found that the most popular activity that most people engaged in is socializing with family and friends. In this context, the study also found a *decreasing marginal utility* of this type activity. That is, to ensure an optimal level of life satisfaction, people attempt to engage in a variety of activities because satisfaction from one type of activity diminishes in time. Sheldon and Niemiec (2006) demonstrated that life balance is achieved not only by the fulfilment of psychological needs (needs for autonomy, competence, and relatedness) but a *balanced effect among the satisfaction of these needs*. Matuska (2012) conceptualized life balance as congruence among both desired and actual time spent in activities and equivalence in the degree of

---

This chapter is adapted partly from Sirgy and Lee (2018b).

© Springer Nature Switzerland AG 2020
M. J. Sirgy, *Positive Balance*, Social Indicators Research Series 80,
https://doi.org/10.1007/978-3-030-40289-1_4

discrepancy between desired and actual time spent across *activities that satisfy basic and growth needs* (needs related to health, relationship, challenge/interest, and identity). This author was able to demonstrate a strong association between life balance and personal well-being. A similar conceptualization was introduced by Sheldon, Cummins, and Kamble (2010). They defined life balance as perceived low discrepancy between actual and ideal time-use profiles. These authors developed a life balance measure based on this conceptualization and were able to demonstrate that life balance is positively related to subjective well-being mediated by psychological need satisfaction.

I tried to address the concept of the balanced life in my 2002 book on the *Psychology of Quality of Life* (Sirgy, 2002). In Chap. 14 of the book, titled "balance," I proposed that people make attempts to create balance in their lives to *optimize* life satisfaction (i.e., achieve and maintain an acceptable level of life satisfaction). I made a distinction between two balance concepts: within-domain balance and between-domain balance. *Balance within a life dom*ain is achieved by striving to experience both positive and negative affect within a given life domain. Positive affect reflects a reward function, namely goals are attained, and resources are acquired. In contrast, negative affect serves a motivational function. That is, negative affect helps the individual recognize problems and opportunities for future achievement and growth (cf. Kitayama & Markus, 2000). *Balance between life domains* can be achieved through compensation; that is, increasing the salience of positive life domains compensates for negative life domains; and conversely, decreasing the salience of negative life domains helps reduce the influence of negative affect from these domains on overall life satisfaction (also see Sirgy, 2012). I with a doctoral student at the time (Sirgy & Wu, 2009) published an article in the *Journal of Happiness Studies* titled "The pleasant life, the engaged life, and the meaningful life: What about the balanced life?" In that article we positioned the concept of the balanced life vis-à-vis other popular concepts of subjective well-being, namely "the pleasant life," "the engaged life," and "the meaningful life" (as proposed by Martin Seligman in his 2002 book, *Authentic Happiness*). Seligman has argued that life satisfaction stems from three major sets of experiences in life, namely experiencing pleasantness regularly (the pleasant life), experiencing a high level of engagement in satisfying activities (the engaged life), and experiencing a sense of connectedness to a greater whole (the meaningful life). In response, we countered by suggesting that having a balanced life is equally important to life satisfaction. The balanced life is experienced when people are highly engaged in social roles in multiple domains. We explained the effect of balance on life satisfaction using two concepts, namely *satisfaction limits* (people can derive only limited amount of satisfaction from a single life domain; hence engagement in multiple domains is necessary to optimize life satisfaction) and *satisfaction of the full spectrum of human developmental needs* (people have to be involved in multiple domains to satisfy both basic and growth needs; both sets of needs have to be met to induce a high level of subjective well-being). That article won the Best Paper in the journal and was reprinted in *Explorations of Happiness* (edited by Delle Fave, 2013).

As such, in this chapter I offer a definition of positive mental health characteristic of positive balance and discuss three major principles of life balance and describe how life balance in domain satisfaction contributes to subjective well-being (life satisfaction or perceived quality of life). The definition is as follows: *Individuals experiencing a having a preponderance of domain satisfaction (satisfaction in salient and multiple life domains such as family life, work life, social life, etc.) relative to dissatisfaction in other life domains.* Furthermore, the reader could benefit from understanding how the well-being concept at the cognitive level (domain satisfaction) emerges from the concept of well-being at the emotional level (hedonic well-being or positive and negative affect). I argue that this emergence process involves domain segmentation (see Table 4.1).

Life Balance

To follow the subsequent discussion on life balance, the reader needs to become familiar with certain concepts such as domain segmentation, domain satisfaction, and life satisfaction. Andrews and Withey (1976) and Campbell, Converse, and Rodgers (1976) were the main proponents of the life domain approach to the study of domain and life satisfaction. Andrews and Withey used multiple regression to predict subjects' life satisfaction scores ("How do you feel about life as a whole?" with responses captured on a 7-point delighted-terrible scale). They found satisfaction with various life domains explained 52–60% of the variance. Many other quality-of-life/well-being researchers have shown that domain satisfaction contribute significantly accounts for much of the life satisfaction scores (see literature reviews by Diener, 1984; Diener, Suh, Lucas, & Smith, 1999). The notion of satisfaction in life domains contributing to a life satisfaction judgment has come to be known as *bottom-up spillover theory of life satisfaction* (Sirgy, 2012).

Affective experiences are stored in memory in life spheres (or life segments), and these spheres are organized in a hierarchy of satisfaction. At the top of the satisfaction hierarchy is life satisfaction—a hot cognition reflecting how the individual feels about his or her life overall. Second in line in the satisfaction hierarchy is domain satisfaction. That is, people make judgments about how they feel in certain life domains such as family life, social life, work life, material life, community life, etc. Satisfaction in these life domains influences the life satisfaction judgment, which is at the top of the satisfaction hierarchy—the most abstract hot cognition. At the bottom of the satisfaction hierarchy are concrete hot cognitions related to satisfaction with life events (i.e., concrete and salient events that have occurred and are associated with positive or negative affect). As such, satisfaction judgments related to life events (most concrete hot cognitions) influence satisfaction judgments of life domains, which in turn influence satisfaction with life overall (most abstract hot cognition). The reader should then note that the central tenet of bottom-up spillover theory of life satisfaction is the carryover of affect from subordinate life domains to superordinate ones, specifically from life domains such as leisure, family, job, and

Table 4.1 Positive mental health defined at various hierarchical levels as positive balance with emergence and focus on the cognitive level

Level of analysis	Positive balance as positive mental health	Programs of research	Emergence
Positive mental health defined at a physiological level = **positive and negative neurotransmitters**	Individuals experiencing a preponderance of neurochemicals related to positive emotions (dopamine, serotonin, oxytocin) relative to neurochemicals related to negative emotions (cortisol)	Stress response system); neurobiology of happiness)	
Positive mental health defined at an emotional level = **positive/negative affect or hedonic well-being (positive/negative neurotransmitters + cognitive appraisals)**	Individuals experiencing a preponderance of positive emotions (happiness, joy, serenity, contentment, etc.) relative to negative emotions (anger, sadness, jealousy, envy, depression, etc.)	Positive versus negative affect; broaden and build theory; flow	Positive neurochemicals (dopamine, serotonin, and oxytocin) at the physiological level mediated by a process of cognitive appraisal (positive frame) result into positive affect (happiness, joy, contentment, etc.) at the emotional level; and conversely, negative neurochemicals (cortisol) mediated by a process of cognitive appraisal (negative frame) result into negative affect (anger, sadness, jealousy, envy, depression, etc.)
Positive mental health defined at a cognitive level = **domain satisfaction (positive/negative affect + domain segmentation)**	Individuals experiencing a preponderance of domain satisfaction (satisfaction in salient and multiple life domains such as family life, work life, social life, etc.) relative to dissatisfaction in other life domains	Principle of satisfaction limits; principle of the full spectrum of human developmental needs; principle of diminishing satisfaction	Positive affect (happiness, joy, contentment, etc.) at the emotional level mediated by a process of domain segmentation result into domain satisfaction (satisfied with work life, social life, family life, etc.); and conversely, negative affect (anger, sadness, jealousy, envy, depression, etc.) mediated by a process of domain segmentation result into domain dissatisfaction (dissatisfied with work life, social life, family life, etc.)
Positive mental health defined at a meta-cognitive level = **life satisfaction (domain satisfaction + bottom-up process)**	Individuals experiencing a preponderance of positive evaluations about one's life using certain standards of comparison (satisfaction with one's life compared to one's past life, the life of family members, the life of associates at work, the life of others in the same social circles, etc.) relative to negative evaluations about one's life using similar or other standards of comparison	Multiple discrepancies theory; congruity life satisfaction; temporal life satisfaction; social comparison; frequency of positive affect; homeostatically protected mood	Domain satisfaction (satisfied with work life, social life, family life, etc.) at the cognitive level mediated by a bottom-up process at the meta-cognitive level result in life satisfaction; and conversely. domain dissatisfaction (dissatisfied with work life, social life, family life, etc.) mediated by a bottom-up process result in life dissatisfaction

(continued)

Table 4.1 (continued)

Positive mental health defined at a developmental level = **eudaimonia (life satisfaction + personal growth)**	Individuals experiencing a preponderance of positive psychological traits (self-acceptance, personal growth, purpose in life, environmental mastery, autonomy, positive relations with others, etc.) relative to negative psychological traits (pessimism, hopelessness, depressive disorder, neuroticism, impulsiveness, etc.)	Hedonic versus eudaimonic happiness; virtue ethics and character strengths; self-determination theory; personal expressiveness; psychological well-being; purpose and meaning in life; flourishing; orientations to happiness; resilience; and satisfaction of the full spectrum of human needs	Life satisfaction at the meta-cognitive level mediated by a process involving high personal growth result in high levels of eudaimonia at the developmental level; and conversely, life dissatisfaction mediated by a process involving low personal growth result into low levels of eudaimonia
Positive mental health defined at a social-ecological level = **socio-eudaimonia (eudaimonia + social & moral development)**	Individuals experiencing a preponderance of social resources (social acceptance, social actualization, social contribution, social integration, social harmony, social belongingness, social attachment, familial attachment, etc.) relative to social constraints (social alienation, social discord, social exclusion, ostracism, etc.)	Social well-being, social harmony need to belong, attachment theory; social exclusion and ostracism	High levels of eudaimonia at the developmental level mediated by a process involving high social and moral development result into high levels of socio-eudaimonia at the social-ecological level; and conversely, low levels of eudaimonia mediated by a process involving low social and moral development result into low levels of socio-eudaimonia

health to overall life. Thus, bottom-up spillover implies that subjective well-being (or more specifically, life satisfaction) can be increased by allowing life domains carrying positive feelings or satisfaction to spill over unto the most superordinate domain (overall life). The positive affect accumulates in life domains as a direct function of satisfaction of human development needs—physiological needs, safety needs, social needs, esteem needs, self-actualization needs, knowledge needs, and aesthetics needs (Maslow, 1970).

Having explained the concepts of life domains and domain satisfaction, the reader is now ready to appreciate the discussion concerning how people manipulate the interplay life domains and domain satisfaction to increase life balance, which in turn contributes to life satisfaction. That is, to achieve life balance people engage in behavioral strategies to increase life satisfaction by manipulating the interplay among domain satisfaction to prompt greater participation of satisfied life domains and contribute to life satisfaction, namely (1) engagement in social roles in multiple life domains (explained by the principle of satisfaction limits), (2) engagement in roles in health, safety, economic, social, work, leisure, and cultural domains (explained by the principle of satisfaction of the full spectrum of human

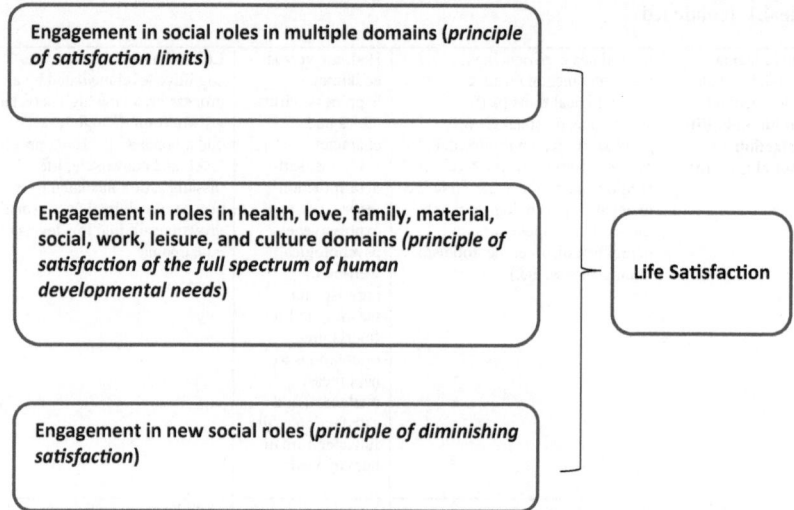

Fig. 4.1 Domain satisfaction strategies people use to create balance

development needs), and (3) engagement in new social roles (explained by the principle of diminishing satisfaction). See Fig. 4.1.

Engagement in Social Roles in Multiple Life Domains and the Principle of Satisfaction Limits

Much research has shown that engagement in social roles in work life and nonwork life (family, leisure, social, community, etc.) serves to produce a positive, fulfilling, state of mind characterized as vigor, dedication, and absorption (Schaufeli, Salanova, Gonzalez-Roma, & Bakker, 2002). *Vigor* reflects a high level of energy and mental resilience in role engagement in multiple domains. *Dedication* refers to being strongly involved in one's roles at both work and nonwork by experiencing a sense of significance, enthusiasm, and challenge. *Absorption* is characterized by being fully concentrated and happily engrossed in the task at hand associated with the various roles across life domains (Schaufeli & Bakker, 2004).

Individuals are likely to achieve a high level of satisfaction in life overall when they are fully engaged in multiple roles in work *and* nonwork life. Further, they are likely to maximize their life satisfaction if and when they become fully engaged in *multiple* roles. Doing so is essentially one way to increase harmony among life domains. Increasing satisfaction in multiple domains ultimately serves to increase life satisfaction at large. The effect of role engagement in social roles in multiple domains on life satisfaction can be explained through the *principle of satisfaction limits,* which we now turn to.

The bottom-up spillover model of life satisfaction proposes that life satisfaction is determined by cumulative satisfaction experienced in important life domains such as satisfaction in work life, family life, social life, leisure life, spiritual life, community life, etc. (e.g., Andrews & Withey, 1976; Campbell et al., 1976). Mathematically speaking, the model states that a life satisfaction score of an individual can be predicted by adding all the satisfaction scores of salient life domains. For example, if one uses an 11-point satisfaction scale (-5 = high dissatisfaction to +5 = high satisfaction), then an individual (A) registering satisfaction in work life (e.g., "+3"), family life (e.g., "+3"), leisure life (e.g., "+3"), social life (e.g., "+3"), and material life (e.g., "+3") should have a higher life satisfaction score than another individual (B) who registers satisfaction in work life (e.g., "+5"), family life (e.g., "0"), leisure life (e.g., "0"), social life (e.g., "0"), and material life (e.g., "0"). This is due to the fact that the former individual has a total domain satisfaction score of "15" [(+3) + (+3) + (+3) + (+3) + (+3)], whereas the latter has a total domain satisfaction score of "+5" [(+5) + (0) + (0) + (0) + (0)]. Of course, this predictive equation assumes that work life, family life, leisure life, social life, and material life are all equally salient to both individuals. In other words, overall life satisfaction is accrued additively from satisfaction in multiple life domains. Research has demonstrated that satisfaction from a variety of life domains contributes to unique variance in life satisfaction, and that there is some validity to this compensatory model of life satisfaction (e.g., Hsieh, 2003; Rojas, 2006; also see reviews by Diener, 1984; Diener et al., 1999).

The *principle of satisfaction limits* (Sirgy & Wu, 2009) posits that the amount of contribution of domain satisfaction from a single life domain to overall life satisfaction is limited. In the example of the compensatory model described above the limit is +5 satisfaction units in each domain (scale = +5 to -5). In other words, one can achieve only a limited amount of satisfaction from a single life domain (a maximum of 5 satisfaction units). Using the example above, Person A is satisfied in work life ("+3"), leisure life ("+3"), social life ("+3"), material life ("+3"), and family life ("+3"). His life satisfaction (15 units) is based on a moderate degree of satisfaction in five salient life domains. Person B is satisfied with work life (+5) only. He is not satisfied in family life ("0"), leisure life ("0"), social life ("0"), as well as material life ("0"). His life satisfaction score ("5" units) is based on satisfaction from 1 out of 5 salient domains. In sum, an individual who is highly satisfied in *multiple domains* is likely to experience a higher life satisfaction compared to an individual who is highly satisfied in a single domain. As such, role engagement in multiple life domains produces an additive effect on life satisfaction (e.g., Andrews & Withey, 1976; Campbell et al., 1976; Eakman, 2016; Hsieh, 2003; Rojas, 2006; Sirgy & Lee, 2016; Sirgy & Wu, 2009). That is, high role engagement in a single life domain with little or no role engagement in other life domains cannot contribute much to life satisfaction compared to high role engagement in multiple domains.

Consider the following study: Bhargava (1995) asked study participants to discuss life satisfaction of others. Most participants inferred life satisfaction of others as a direct function of their satisfaction in *multiple* domains. They calculated happiness by summing satisfaction across several important domains—the more positive affect in multiple domains, the higher the subjective well-being. In a work context, individuals engaging in various social roles in nonwork life domains, in addition to roles in work life, are likely to experience a high level of life satisfaction compared to those who are highly engaged only in work life (e.g., Greenhaus & Powell, 2006; Rice, McFarlin, Hunt, & Near, 1985).

In sum, this discussion can be summarized as follows: Individuals who have a high level of role engagement in multiple life domains are likely to increase life balance and experience higher life satisfaction than those who have a high level of role engagement in a single domain. This effect may be due to satisfaction limits. Specifically, compared to individuals who are engaged in a single domain, individuals who are highly engaged in multiple life domains are likely to experience more satisfaction in those domains, contributing to life satisfaction. Those who are engaged in a single domain can produce only a limited amount of domain satisfaction (less that those who are engaged in multiple domains) that spills over to life satisfaction. That is, compared to role engagement in multiple domains, role engagement in a single domain is likely to be wholly insufficient to contribute significantly to life satisfaction.

Engagement in Roles in Health, Love, Family, Material, Social, Work, Leisure, and Culture Domains; and the Principle of Satisfaction of the Full Spectrum of Human Developmental Needs

People try to optimize their life satisfaction (enhance their life satisfaction to an acceptable level) by actively engaging in social roles in multiple domains. The question that arises based on the preceding argument is "which domains?" Life satisfaction is significantly increased when the individual engages in roles in life domains that can satisfy the full spectrum of human development needs (Maslow, 1970). As such, life balance can be achieved through active engagement in social roles in multiple domains serving to satisfy *both* basic and growth needs: health, love, family, and material domains serving to satisfy mostly basic needs; and social, work, leisure, and culture domains serving to satisfy growth needs. Let us be more specific.

Sirgy and Wu (2009) have argued that subjective well-being is not simply cumulative positive minus negative affect—irrespective of the source. It is the satisfaction of human developmental needs, the full range of needs—not a handful of selected needs. In other words, one cannot substitute positive affect related to one need with another need. To illustrate this point, let us consider the following example. Two individuals, A and B. Person A has "+3" satisfaction units in each of the following domains related to basic needs: health life, love life, family life, and material life. In other words, Person A is satisfied in domains related to his basic needs, a total score of "+8" satisfaction units [(+2) + (+2) + (+2) + (+2)] and the same person is similarly satisfied in life domains related to growth needs (social life, work life, leisure life, and culture life), a total of "+8" [(+2) + (+2) + (+2) + (+2)]. Summing up Person A's domain satisfaction scores, we obtain a total amount of "16" units of domain satisfaction (+8 satisfaction units from domains related to basic needs, and another +8 satisfaction units from domains related to growth needs). Now let us compare this case with Person B who is highly satisfied with basic needs only. Person B is highly satisfied in domains related to his basic needs, a total score of "+20" satisfaction units [(+5) + (+5) + (+5) + (+5)] while is dissatisfied in domains related to his growth needs, a total of "−8" satisfaction units [(−2) + (−2) + (−2) + (−2)]. As such, the total domain satisfaction score for person B is also "+12". We predict that person A is likely to report a higher degree of life satisfaction than person B because person A has *balanced satisfaction* from life domains related to *both basic and growth needs*, whereas Person B has unbalanced domain satisfaction (high satisfaction in domains related to basic needs but low satisfaction in domains related to growth needs).

Let us delve deeper to understand the psychology underling this effect. Let's do so by discussing the *principle of satisfaction of the full spectrum of human developmental needs*. This principle posits that individuals who are satisfied with the full spectrum of developmental needs (i.e., satisfaction of growth needs as well as basic needs) are likely to have a high level of life satisfaction relative to those who are less satisfied (e.g., Alderfer, 1972; Herzberg, 1966; Maslow, 1970; Matuska, 2012; Sheldon et al., 2010; Sheldon & Niemiec, 2006). When people engage in multiple roles across life domains, they are likely to obtain access to psychological and physical resources, which in turn increase opportunities for satisfaction of many basic and growth needs. Seeking to satisfy a specific need in a single life domain does not positively contribute much to life satisfaction (Sirgy et al., 1995). That is, when people engage in multiple roles, they are likely to experience satisfaction of growth needs (i.e., social, knowledge, aesthetics, self-actualization, and self-transcendence needs) as well as satisfaction of basic needs (i.e., health, safety, and economic needs). Satisfaction of growth needs contributes to positive affect, whereas satisfaction of basic needs contributes mostly to the reduction of negative affect (Herzberg, 1966). Satisfaction of both sets of basic and growth needs contributes significantly and positively to life satisfaction.

Specifically, Sirgy and Wu (2009) have described how people organize their lives to fulfil their developmental needs. To satisfy their biological and health-related needs, people engage in a variety of activities such as eating right, exercising regularly, getting regular check-ups, engaging in regular sex, and so on. The events related to those activities and their outcomes generate a certain amount of satisfaction and dissatisfaction. These affective reactions are organized and stored in memory in certain life domains such as health, love, family, and economic. When a man is asked how he feels about his health life, he is likely to reflect on his affective experiences in relation to health-related activities such as eating right, exercising regularly, having regular check-ups, and so on. When the same person is asked about his love life, he reflects about his affective experiences related to love, romantic relationships, and sex. When asked about his family life, he reflects on those experiences related to the use of his significant others such as spouse and children, his residence, his neighborhood, and community. Financial issues and experiences related to money, income, standard of living, and material possessions also likely to be segmented in material life and mostly related to basic needs. With respect to growth needs (e.g., social, esteem, self-actualization, self-transcendence, aesthetics, and knowledge needs), experiences may be segmented in life domains such as social life, work life, leisure life, and culture life. However, this is not to say that a variety of developmental needs can be met in a single domain. Consider the work domain for example. Many developmental needs, both basic and growth needs, can be met through work life. Through work life, both basic (i.e., economic, health and safety, and family-related needs) and growth needs (i.e., social, esteem, self-actualization, self-transcendence, knowledge, and aesthetics needs) can be met. To reiterate, in every life domain a variety of developmental needs can be met. However, certain life domains are predisposed to meet certain developmental needs more so than others. As such, health, love, family, and economic domains are likely to reflect satisfaction resulting more from meeting basic than growth needs. Conversely, social life, work life, leisure life, and culture life are domains likely to reflect satisfaction resulting more from meeting growth than basic needs.

Suggestive evidence of this principle comes from a body of evidence showing that materialism is negatively correlated with life satisfaction (see Wright & Larsen, 1993, for a meta-analysis of the research findings). Specifically, materialistic people can be viewed as imbalanced in that they pursue wealth and material possessions to the exclusion of other important goals in life. Materialistic people who are successful hoarding material wealth may feel successful and happy with their material life. Placing undue emphasis on making money (to satisfy basic needs such as biological and safety needs) is likely to lead them to neglect other growth needs such as social, esteem, self-actualization, self-transcendence, aesthetics, and knowledge needs. It is no wonder that the evidence shows that materialism is negatively correlated with life satisfaction.

Furthermore, as previously discussed, Matuska (2012) conceptualized life balance as congruence among both desired and actual time spent in activities and equivalence in the degree of discrepancy between desired and actual time spent across *activities that satisfy basic and growth needs* (needs related to health, relationship, challenge/interest, and identity). The author conducted a study that successfully demonstrated a strong association between life balance and personal well-being.

In sum, the preceding discussion can be summarized as follows: Individuals who have a high level of role engagement in life domains related to both basic needs (e.g., health, love, family, and material domains) and growth needs (e.g., social, work, leisure, and culture domains) are likely to experience greater satisfaction among life domains contributing to higher life satisfaction than those who have a high level of role engagement in domains related to only basic or growth needs. This effect may be due to the effect of satisfaction of the full spectrum of human developmental needs. Specifically, compared to individuals who are engaged in roles in select domains, individuals who have a high level of role engagement in multiple domains addressing both basic and growth needs are likely to experience more life satisfaction. Role engagement in health, love, family, and material domains are likely to satisfy mostly basic needs (survival needs such as having enough resources to deal with health and safety issues), whereas role engagement in social, work, leisure, and culture are likely to satisfy mostly growth needs (higher-order needs such as social, esteem, self-actualization, aesthetics, and knowledge needs). The combined and balanced effects of satisfaction of both basic and growth needs serve to increase life satisfaction. That is, satisfaction of the full spectrum of human developmental needs (balance between basic and growth need satisfaction) produce the highest level of life satisfaction.

Engagement in New Social Roles and the Principle of Diminishing Satisfaction

Much research in variety seeking supports the notion that successful engagement in new roles is likely to produce more positive affect than successful engagement in well-established roles (e.g., Kahn, 1995; Kahn & Isen, 1993; Levav & Zhu, 2009; McAlister & Pessemier, 1982). That is, engaging and succeeding in new roles tend to produce a jolt of positive affect much more so than engaging and succeeding in well-established roles. Also, much research in industrial/organizational (I/O) psychology has demonstrated the effect of task variety on job performance and employee well-being (e.g., Christian, Garza, & Slaughter, 2011; Pierce & Dunham, 1976). That is, compared to workers who are engaged in repetitive tasks, workers engaging in a variety of tasks tend to feel much more motivated to excel on their jobs, tend to do much better in relation to job performance, and experience higher levels of job satisfaction. One can extrapolate from this research that life balance is not only limited to engagement in social roles in multiple domains satisfying both basic and growth-related needs but also new social roles. This may best be explained using the *principle of diminishing satisfaction.*

This principle states that individuals with life balance are likely to continuously engage in new roles to guard against diminishing satisfaction associated with well-established roles. Why? The intensity of the positive affect in the context of a social role experienced in a given life domain tends to decay with adaptation effects (Helson, 1964). Consider the following scenarios. Person A (woman) is right out of college and starts a new job. She experiences success in her assigned roles. This success is likely to bring much positive affect and satisfaction in work life— +4 units of satisfaction in the work domain—on a 11-point satisfaction scale varying from −5 (very dissatisfied) to +5 (very satisfied). Compare Person A (woman) to Person B (man) who is a seasoned worker—has been on the job for a long time. He is equally successful in his assigned work roles (perhaps a +2 units of satisfaction). That is, the man is not likely to experience the same magnitude of satisfaction compared to the woman. This dampening of positive affect and satisfaction for the man is due to an adaptation effect. That is, positive affect is dampened with repeated successful performance. To guard against this dampening effect and to restore satisfaction in the work life domain, the man must engage in new roles to maintain the same level of domain satisfaction that was once generated through old and well-established role performance. However, to increase positive affect in the work domain (say from +2 units of satisfaction to +4 units of satisfaction), he needs to engage in new work-related roles successfully.

Research has documented this phenomenon. Specifically, given successful role performance in a particular life domain (e.g., work life) individuals who have not been feeling satisfied in that domain are likely to experience a greater magnitude of domain satisfaction than individuals who are already satisfied in the same domain (e.g., Ahuvia & Friedman, 1998; Diener et al., 2008; Rojas, 2006). Put succinctly, increases in satisfaction in a life domain serve to increase life satisfaction but at a decreasing marginal rate with repeated experiences.

In sum, we can capture the preceding discussion as follows: Individuals become engaged in new social roles to mitigate decreases in domain satisfaction and life satisfaction overall. This effect is due to the diminishing satisfaction effect. Specifically, individuals who are engaged in social roles experience diminishing satisfaction in a given life domain over time, which in turn detract from life satisfaction overall. To guard against this diminishing domain satisfaction, they engage in new social roles to generate new satisfaction thereby compensating for the diminished satisfaction related to the old roles.

Emergence[1]

How does well-being at the emotional level (hedonic well-being) impact the formation and maintenance of well-being at the cognitive level (domain satisfaction)? As argued in the last chapter, this link can be viewed in terms of emergence—a concept well-entrenched in systems science. To reiterate, emergence refers to higher-level systems "emerge" from lower-level systems. The research related to positive and negative affect leads us to a clear conclusion. This conclusion is captured as follows: in the following theoretical proposition: *Positive affect (happiness, joy, contentment, etc.) at the emotional level moderated by domain segmentation result into domain satisfaction (satisfied with work life, social life, family life, etc.); and conversely, negative affect (anger, sadness, jealousy, envy, depression, etc.) mediated by a process of domain segmentation result into domain dissatisfaction (dissatisfied with work life, social life, family life, etc.).* See Fig. 4.2.

As previously mentioned, Andrews and Withey (1976) and Campbell et al. (1976) are the main proponents of the life domain approach to the study of well-being. For example, Andrews and Withey used multiple regression to predict

---

[1]This section has been partly adapted from Sirgy (2012, Chap. 16).

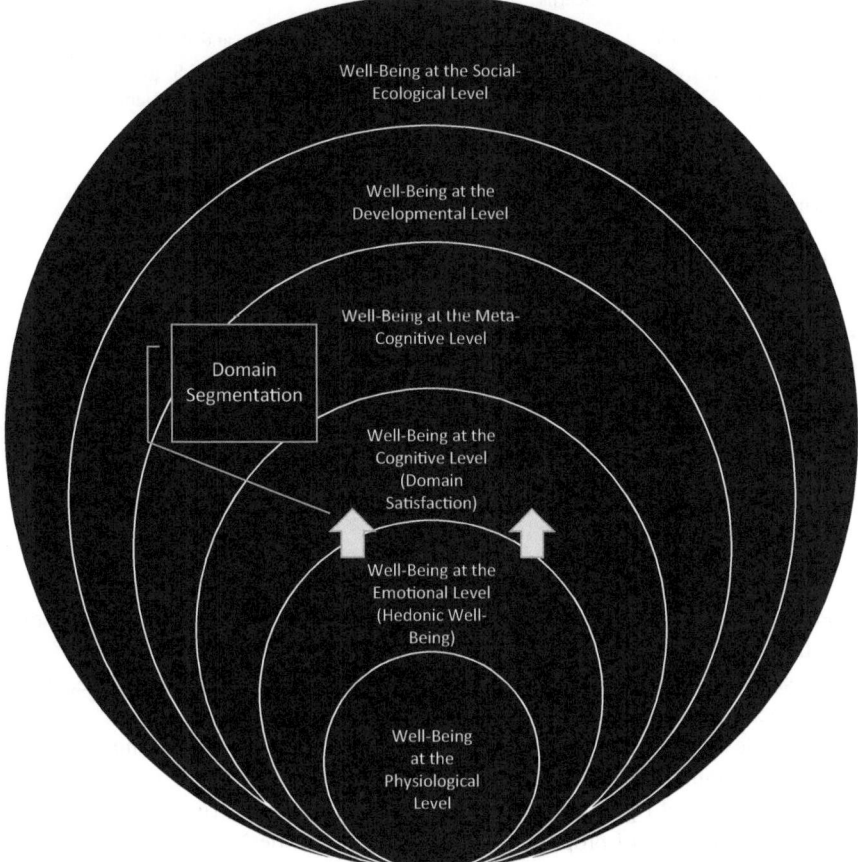

Fig. 4.2 Emergence: well-being at the cognitive level (domain satisfaction) influenced by well-being at the emotional level (hedonic well-being) mediated by a process of domain segmentation

subjects' life satisfaction scores ("How do you feel about life as a whole?" with responses captured on a 7-point delighted-terrible scale). They found that satisfaction with various life domains (see Table 4.2) explained from 52 to 60% of the variance.

Based on a synthesis of the health-related quality-of-life literature, Schalock (1996) was able to identify life domains that seem to play a significant role in well-being. These are:

- Emotional and psychological well-being (i.e., safety, spirituality, happiness, contentment, freedom from stress),
- Interpersonal and social relationships (i.e., family well-being, friendships, intimate relationships, supportive network),
- Material well-being (i.e., income, financial security, material possessions, savings and investments, meeting basic needs such as food and shelter),

Table 4.2 Domains of life concerns

Campbell et al. (1976)	Andrews and Withey (1976)
• Non-working activities	• Life in the U.S. today
• Family life	• National government
• Standard of living	• Local government
• Work	• Economic situation
• Marriage	• Community
• Savings and investments	• Services and facilities
• Friendships	• Education
• City or county	• Jobs
• Housing	• Neighbourhood
• Amount of education	• Friends and associates
• Neighbourhood	• Home
• Life in the U.S.	• Leisure and leisure-time activities
• Usefulness of education	• Family
• Health	• Self
• Religion	• Interpersonal relations
• National government	
• Organisations	

Source: Adapted from Day (1987, p. 16)

- Personal development (i.e., competence, educational attainment, purposeful activities, mastery, effectance, achievements and goal attainment),
- Physical well-being (i.e., health and wellness, nutrition, physical exercise, sports and recreation, activities related to daily living),
- Social development (i.e., inclusion in the community, volunteering activities, charity, neighborhood cohesion), and
- Civic duties and rights (i.e., privacy rights, voting rights, right to due process, right to ownership of property, and civic responsibilities).

Furthermore, instruments developed by the WHOQOL Group (1998, 2004, 2006) use the following 11 life domains, well-established in the health and well-being literature:

- work,
- family,
- standard of living,
- interpersonal relationships,
- health,
- personal growth,
- spirituality/religion,
- society issues,
- community issues,
- leisure, and
- life in general.

Cummins (1996) identified 1500 articles related to life satisfaction and investigated the life domains that these authors have focused on. Altogether, Cummins selected 32 studies using at least two screening criteria: the article must have at least three domains representing well-being or quality of life, and the article must have a detailed description of the measures used and average scores of each domain. These studies collectively named 351 different domain names. Using factor analytic techniques, Cummins was able to identify seven major key domains that accounted for most of the variance. These are:

- material well-being,
- health,
- productivity,
- intimacy,
- safety,
- community, and
- emotional well-being.

In their recent book, *Well Being: The Five Essential Elements*, Tom Rath and Jim Harter (2010) of the Gallup organization report the five most important life domains that impact well-being the most are:

- career life,
- social life,
- financial life,
- physical/health life, and
- community life.

These findings are based on "hundreds of questions across countries, languages, and vastly different life situations" (p. 5). Career well-being is about how a person occupies his or her time or simply what that person likes what they do every day. Social well-being is about strong relationships and love in a person's life. Financial well-being is about effectively managing one's economic situation and personal finances. Physical well-being is about having good health and enough energy to get things done on a daily basis. Finally, community well-being is about the sense of engagement one has with the area he or she resides.

Van Praag and Ferrer-I-Carbonell (2010), in a review special issue of *Foundations and Trends in Microeconomics*, addressed the aggregation of domain satisfaction in relation to life satisfaction. The following results are presented in the book authored by Van Praag and Ferrer-I-Carbonell (2004, 2008) on *Happiness Quantified*. These results indicate that for working people the sense of well-being (domain satisfaction) in relation to work is equally important to social well-being, which is closely followed by health well-being and leisure-use well-being. For non-workers (i.e., students, retired people, housewives, and the unemployed), too much leisure may be detrimental to life satisfaction.

Much of this discussion point to the notion that people segment their positive and negative feelings concerning life events in "life domains." This is what I am calling "domain segmentation." As such, people do not have difficulty responding to survey questions about their various domains (work life, family life, love life, social life, leisure life, etc.). This type of domain segmentation allows them to articulate the perceived positive and negative affect stowed away in these various domains. As such, based on the preceding discussion, I am fairly confident of the emergence proposition I fleshed out at the beginning of this section, namely that *positive affect (happiness, joy, contentment, etc.) at the emotional level is mediated by a process of domain segmentation resulting into domain satisfaction (satisfied with work life, social life, family life, etc.); and conversely, negative affect (anger, sadness, jealousy, envy, depression, etc.) is mediated by a process of domain segmentation resulting into domain dissatisfaction (dissatisfied with work life, social life, family life, etc.)* (Fig. 4.2).

Conclusion

The research involving these three principles (the principle of satisfaction limits, the principle of the full spectrum of human developmental needs, and the principle of diminishing satisfaction) support my definition of positive balance at the cognitive level. That is, positive mental health at the cognitive level can be defined as: Individuals characterized as having positive mental health tend to experience a preponderance of domain satisfaction (satisfaction in salient and multiple life domains such as family life, work life, social life, etc.) relative to dissatisfaction in other life domains. I also argued that positive affect at the emotional level, mediated by a process of domain segmentation, result into domain satisfaction; and conversely, negative affect, mediated by a process of domain segmentation, result into domain dissatisfaction.

The next chapter will focus on positive balance as viewed from the meta-cognitive level of analysis. I will focus on the concept of life satisfaction and show that domain satisfaction (well-being at the cognitive level) plays an important role in the "emergence" of well-being at that meta-cognitive level, namely life satisfaction. A definition of positive balance at the meta-cognitive level will be discussed with supportive evidence from several programs of research: multiple discrepancies theory, congruity life satisfaction, temporal life satisfaction, social comparison, frequency of positive affect, and homeostatically protected mood.

References

Ahuvia, A. C., & Friedman, D. C. (1998). Income, consumption, and subjective well-being: Toward a composite macromarketing model. *Journal of Macromarketing, 18*, 153–168.

Alderfer, C. P. (1972). *Existence, relatedness, and growth: Human needs in organizational settings.* New York: Free Press.

Allen, T. D., Herst, D. E., Bruck, C. S., & Sutton, M. (2000). Consequences associated with work-to-family conflict: A review and agenda for future research. *Journal of Occupational Health Psychology, 5*, 278–308.

Andrews, F. M., & Withey, S. B. (1976). *Social indicators of well-being: America's perception of life quality.* New York: Plenum.

Bhargava, S. (1995). An integration-theoretical analysis of life satisfaction. *Psychological Studies, 40,* 170–187.

Bulger, C. A., & Fisher, G. G. (2012). Ethical imperatives of work/life balance. In N. P. Reilly, M. J. Sirgy, & C. A. Gorman (Eds.), *Work and quality of life* (pp. 181–202). Dordrecht: Springer.

Byron, K. (2005). A meta-analytic review of work-family conflict and its antecedents. *Journal of Vocational Behavior, 67,* 169–198.

Campbell, A., Converse, P. E., & Rodgers, W. L. (1976). *The quality of American life: Perceptions, evaluations, and satisfactions.* New York: Russell Sage Foundation.

Casper, W. J., Eby, L. T., Bordeaux, C., Lockwood, A., & Lambert, D. (2007). A review of research methods in IO/OB work family research. *Journal of Applied Psychology, 92,* 28–43.

Christian, M. S., Garza, A. S., & Slaughter, J. E. (2011). Work engagement: A quantitative review and test of its relations with task and contextual performance. *Personnel Psychology, 64,* 89–136.

Cummins, R. A. (1996). The domains of life satisfaction: An attempt to order chaos. *Social Indicators Research, 38,* 303–332.

Danna, K., & Griffin, R. W. (1999). Health and well-being in the workplace: A review and synthesis of the literature. *Journal of Management, 25,* 357–384.

Day, R. L. (1987). Relationship between life satisfaction and consumer satisfaction. In A. C. Samli (Ed.), *Marketing and quality-of-life interface* (pp. 289–311). Westport, CT: Greenwood Press.

Delle Fave, A. (Ed.). (2013). *The exploration of happiness: Present and future perspectives.* Dordrecht: Springer.

Diener, E. (1984). Subjective well-being. *Psychological Bulletin, 75,* 542–575.

Diener, E., Ng, W., & Tov, W. (2008). Balance in life and declining marginal utility of diverse resources. *Applied Research in Quality of Life, 3,* 277–291.

Diener, E., Suh, E., Lucas, R., & Smith, H. (1999). Subjective well-being: Three decades of research. *Psychological Bulletin, 125,* 276–302.

Eakman, A. M. (2016). A subjectively-based definition of life balance using personal meaning in occupation. *Journal of Occupational Science, 23,* 108–127.

Eby, L. T., Casper, W. J., Lockwood, A., Bordeaux, C., & Brinley, A. (2005). Work and family research in IO/OB: Content analysis and review of the literature (1980–2002). *Journal of Vocational Behavior, 66,* 124–197.

Eby, L. T., Maher, C. P., & Butts, M. M. (2010). The intersection of work and family life: The role of affect. *Annual Review of Psychology, 61,* 599–622.

Greenhaus, J. H., & Allen, T. D. (2011). Work-family balance: A review and extension of the literature. In J. C. Quick & L. E. Tetrick (Eds.), *Handbook of occupational health psychology* (2nd ed., pp. 165–183). Washington, DC: American Psychological Association.

Greenhaus, J. H., & Powell, G. N. (2006). When work and family are allies: A theory of work-family enrichment. *Academy of Management Review, 31,* 72–92.

Helson, H. (1964). Current trends and issues in adaptation-level theory. *American Psychologist, 19,* 26–39.

Herzberg, F. (1966). *Work and the nature of man.* Cleveland: World.

Hsieh, C. M. (2003). Counting importance: The case of life satisfaction and relative domain importance. *Social Indicators Research, 61,* 227–240.

Kahn, B. E. (1995). Consumer variety-seeking among goods and services: An integrative review. *Journal of Retailing and Consumer Services, 2,* 139–148.

Kahn, B. E., & Isen, A. M. (1993). The influence of positive affect on variety seeking among safe, enjoyable products. *Journal of Consumer Research, 22,* 257–270.

Kalliath, T., & Brough, P. (2008). Work-life balance: A review of the meaning of the balance construct. *Journal of Management and Organization, 14,* 323–327.

Kitayama, S., & Markus, H. R. (2000). The pursuit of happiness and the realization of sympathy: Cultural patterns of self, social relations, and well-being. In E. Diener & E. M. Suh (Eds.), *Culture and subjective well-being* (pp. 113–161). Cambridge, MA: MIT.

Kossek, E. E., & Ozeki, C. (1998). Work–family conflict, policies, and the job–life satisfaction relationship: A review and directions for organizational behavior–human resources research. *Journal of Applied Psychology, 83*, 139–155.

Lee, D.-J., & Sirgy, M. J. (2017). What do people do to achieve work-life balance? A formative conceptualization to help develop a metric for large-scale quality-of-life surveys. *Social Indicators Research*. Published online.

Levav, J., & Zhu, R. (2009). Seeking freedom through variety. *Journal of Consumer Research, 36*, 600–610.

Maslow, A. H. (1970, 1954). *Motivation and personality*. New York: Harper.

Matuska, K. (2012). Validity evidence of a model and measure of life balance. *Occupation, Participation and Health, 32*, 229–237.

McAlister, L., & Pessemier, E. (1982). Variety seeking behaviour: An interdisciplinary review. *Journal of Consumer Research, 8*, 311–322.

McNall, L. A., Nicklin, J. M., & Masuda, A. D. (2010). A meta-analytic review of the consequences associated with work–family enrichment. *Journal of Business and Psychology, 25*, 381–396.

Pierce, J. L., & Dunham, R. B. (1976). Task design: A literature review. *Academy of Management Review, 1*, 83–97.

Rath, T., & Harter, J. (2010). *Well-being: The five essential elements*. New York: Gallup Press.

Rice, R. W., McFarlin, D. B., Hunt, R. G., & Near, J. P. (1985). Organizational work and the perceived quality of life: Toward a conceptual model. *Academy of Management Review, 10*, 296–310.

Rojas, M. (2006). Life satisfaction and satisfaction in domains of life: Is it a simple or a simplified relationship? *Journal of Happiness Studies, 7*, 467–497.

Schalock, R. (1996). *Quality of life. Volume 1: Conceptualization and measurement*. Washington, DC: American Association on Mental Retardation.

Schaufeli, W. B., & Bakker, A. B. (2004). Job demands, job resources and their relationship with burnout and engagement: A multi-sample study. *Journal of Organizational Behavior, 25*, 293–315.

Schaufeli, W. B., Salanova, M., Gonzalez-Roma, V., & Bakker, A. B. (2002). The measurement of engagement and burnout and: A confirmatory analytic approach. *Journal of Happiness Studies, 3*, 71–92.

Seligman, M. E. P. (2002). *Authentic happiness: Using the new positive psychology to realize your potential for lasting fulfilment*. New York: Free Press.

Sheldon, K. M., Cummins, R., & Kamble, S. (2010). Life balance and well-being: Testing a novel conceptual and measurement approach. *Journal of Personality, 78*, 1093–1134.

Sheldon, K. M., & Niemiec, C. P. (2006). It's not just the amount that counts: Balanced need satisfaction also affects well-being. *Journal of Personality and Social Psychology, 91*, 331–341.

Sirgy, M. J. (2002). *The psychology of quality of life*. Dordrecht: Kluwer Academic.

Sirgy, M. J. (2012). *The psychology of quality of life: Hedonic well-being, life satisfaction, and eudaimonia*. Dordrecht: Springer.

Sirgy, M. J., Cole, D., Kosenko, R., Meadow, H. L., Rahtz, D., Cicic, M., et al. (1995). Developing a life satisfaction measure based on need hierarchy theory. In M. J. Sirgy & A. C. Samli (Eds.), *New dimensions of marketing and quality of life* (pp. 3–26). Westport, CT: Greenwood Press.

Sirgy, M. J., & Lee, D.-J. (2016). Work-life balance: A quality-of-life model. *Applied Research in Quality of Life, 11*, 1059–1082.

Sirgy, M. J., & Lee, D.-J. (2018a). Work-life balance: An integrative review. *Applied Research in Quality of Life,13*, 229–254.

Sirgy, M. J, & Lee, D.-J. (2018b). The psychology of life balance. In E. Diener, S. Oishi, & L. Tay (Eds.), *e-Handbook of well-being, Noba scholar handbook series: Subjective well-being*. Salt Lake City, UT: DEF. nobascholar.com.

Sirgy, M. J., Reilly, N., Wu, J., & Efraty, D. (2008). A work-life identity model of well-being: Towards a research agenda linking quality-of-work-life (QWL) programs with quality of life (QOL). *Applied Research in Quality of Life, 3,* 181–202.

Sirgy, M. J., & Wu, J. (2009). The pleasant life, the engaged life, and the meaningful life: What about the balanced life? *Journal of Happiness Studies, 10,* 183–196.

Van Praag, B. M. S., & Ferrer-I-Carbonell, A. (2004). *Happiness quantified: A satisfaction calculus approach.* New York: Oxford University Press.

Van Praag, B. M. S., & Ferrer-I-Carbonell, A. (2008). *Happiness quantified: A satisfaction calculus approach* (revised ed.). New York: Oxford University Press.

Van Praag, B. M. S., & Ferrer-I-Carbonell, A. (2010). Happiness economics: A new road to measuring and comparing happiness. *Foundations and Trends in Microeconomics, 6,* 1–97.

WHOQOL Group. (1998). The WHOQOL assessment instrument: Development and general psychometric properties. *Social Science and Medicine, 46,* 1585–1596.

WHOQOL Group. (2004). Can we identify the poorest quality of life? Assessing the importance of quality of life using the WHOQOL-100. *Quality of Life Research, 13,* 23–24.

WHOQOL Group. (2006). A cross-cultural study of spirituality, religion, and personal beliefs as components of quality of life. *Social Science and Medicine, 62,* 1486–1497.

Wright, N. D., & Larsen, V. (1993). Materialism and life satisfaction: A meta-analysis. *Journal of Consumer Satisfaction, Dissatisfaction, and Complaining Behavior, 6,* 5–27.

Yasbek, P. (2004). *The business case for firm-level work-life-balance policies: A review of the literature. Labor market policy group.* Wellington: Department of Labour. http://www.dol.govt.nz/PDFs/FirmLevelWLB.pdf

Chapter 5
Positive Balance at the Meta-cognitive Level: Life Satisfaction

Introduction

> The happiness of your life depends upon the quality of your thoughts: therefore, guard accordingly, and take care that you entertain no notions unsuitable to virtue and reasonable nature.—Marcus Aurelius (https://www.brainyquote.com/quotes/marcus_aurelius_121534?src=t_happiness)

Life satisfaction is a concept that has been well-documented in the literature of quality-of-life studies and well-being research; see an extensive description of this concept and related research in much of the research by Diener and his colleagues (see literature review Diener, 1984; Diener, Suh, Lucas, & Smith, 1999). Life satisfaction is one of the four dimensions of subjective well-being. The other three are domain satisfaction, preponderance of positive over negative affect, and the absence of feelings of ill-being. Life satisfaction involves a cognitive evaluation of one's own life. Many large-scale social surveys use the following item to capture life satisfaction: "How satisfied or dissatisfied are you with your life overall? Very dissatisfied (1), Somewhat dissatisfied (2), So/so (3), Somewhat satisfied (4), and Very satisfied (5)." See examples of life satisfaction metrics in Sirgy (2012, Chap. 1 and Appendix). Each of these constructs is distinct although measures of these constructs often correlate substantially, suggesting the need for a higher-order construct.

I argue in this chapter that life satisfaction is essentially an evaluation that an individual makes about his or her life at large, and that this evaluation is a judgment which is strongly influenced by the type of cognitive frame used in decision-making (i.e., standard of comparisons or cognitive referents). That is, the individual judges his or her life against some standard (Day, 1987). This standard of comparison is selected and defined by the individual. It may involve a comparison of one's current life circumstance with old circumstances, a comparison of current life experience with prior expectations, etc. As such, I offer a definition of positive mental health characteristic of positive balance and discuss six programs of research (multiple discrepancies, congruity life satisfaction, temporal life satisfaction, social

© Springer Nature Switzerland AG 2020
M. J. Sirgy, *Positive Balance*, Social Indicators Research Series 80,
https://doi.org/10.1007/978-3-030-40289-1_5

comparison, frequency of positive affect, and homeostatically protected mood) supporting my definition. The definition is as follows: *Individuals characterized as having positive mental health tend to experience a preponderance of positive evaluations about one's life using certain standards of comparison (satisfaction with one's life compared to one's past life, the life of family members, the life of associates at work, the life of others in the same social circles, etc.) relative to negative evaluations about one's life using similar or other standards of comparison.* Following this discussion, the case of emergence is then made. That is, the reader is likely to appreciate the concepts of well-being at the meta-cognitive level by understanding how the concept of life satisfaction is emergent from domain satisfaction. I argue that the concept life satisfaction builds on the concept of domain satisfaction. Domain satisfaction goes through a bottom-up spillover process producing the phenomenon we call life satisfaction. See Table 5.1.

Programs of Research Supporting the Positive Balance Definition

This section of the chapter will cover at least seven research programs and theoretical frameworks that provide support to my definition of positive mental health at the meta-cognitive level. The programs of research are multiple discrepancies theory; congruity life satisfaction; temporal life satisfaction; social comparison; frequency of positive affect; homeostatically protected mood.

Multiple Discrepancies

A widely accepted theory related to how individuals make life satisfaction judgments is *multiple discrepancies theory* (Michalos, 1985, 1986; Michalos et al., 2007). The theory posits that overall life satisfaction is inversely proportional to the perceived differences between what one has versus seven different standards of comparisons. These are:

1. What one wants
2. What others have
3. The best one has had in the past
4. What one expected to have 3 years ago
5. What one expects to have in 5 years
6. What one deserves
7. What one needs

   Michalos (1985) has effectively argued that these standards of comparisons that people use in making life satisfaction judgments are grounded on much theory and

Table 5.1 Positive mental health defined at various hierarchical levels as positive balance with emergence and focus on the meta-cognitive level

Level of analysis	Positive balance as positive mental health	Programs of research	Emergence
Positive mental health defined at a physiological level = **positive and negative neurotransmitters**	Individuals experiencing a preponderance of neurochemicals related to positive emotions (dopamine, serotonin, oxytocin) relative to neurochemicals related to negative emotions (cortisol)	Stress response system); neurobiology of happiness)	
Positive mental health defined at an emotional level = **positive/negative affect or hedonic well-being (positive/negative neurotransmitters + cognitive appraisals)**	Individuals experiencing a preponderance of positive emotions (happiness, joy, serenity, contentment, etc.) relative to negative emotions (anger, sadness, jealousy, envy, depression, etc.)	Positive versus negative affect; broaden and build theory; flow	Positive neurochemicals (dopamine, serotonin, and oxytocin) at the physiological level mediated by a process of cognitive appraisal (positive frame) result into positive affect (happiness, joy, contentment, etc.) at the emotional level; and conversely, negative neurochemicals (cortisol) mediated by a process of cognitive appraisal (negative frame) result into negative affect (anger, sadness, jealousy, envy, depression, etc.)
Positive mental health defined at a cognitive level = **domain satisfaction (positive/negative affect + domain segmentation)**	Individuals experiencing a preponderance of domain satisfaction (satisfaction in salient and multiple life domains such as family life, work life, social life, etc.) relative to dissatisfaction in other life domains	Principle of satisfaction limits; principle of the full spectrum of human developmental needs; principle of diminishing satisfaction	Positive affect (happiness, joy, contentment, etc.) at the emotional level mediated by a process of domain segmentation result into domain satisfaction (satisfied with work life, social life, family life, etc.); and conversely, negative affect (anger, sadness, jealousy, envy, depression, etc.) mediated by a process of domain segmentation result into domain dissatisfaction (dissatisfied with work life, social life, family life, etc.)
Positive mental health defined at a meta-cognitive level = **life satisfaction (domain satisfaction + bottom-up process)**	Individuals experiencing a preponderance of positive evaluations about one's life using certain standards of comparison (satisfaction with one's life compared to one's past life, the life of family members, the life of associates at work, the life of others in the same social circles, etc.) relative to negative evaluations about one's life using similar or other standards of comparison	Multiple discrepancies theory; congruity life satisfaction; temporal life satisfaction; social comparison; frequency of positive affect; homeostatically protected mood	Domain satisfaction (satisfied with work life, social life, family life, etc.) at the cognitive level mediated by a bottom-up process at the meta-cognitive level result in life satisfaction; and conversely. domain dissatisfaction (dissatisfied with work life, social life, family life, etc.) mediated by a bottom-up process result in life dissatisfaction

(continued)

Table 5.1 (continued)

Positive mental health defined at a developmental level = **eudaimonia (life satisfaction + personal growth)**	Individuals experiencing a preponderance of positive psychological traits (self-acceptance, personal growth, purpose in life, environmental mastery, autonomy, positive relations with others, etc.) relative to negative psychological traits (pessimism, hopelessness, depressive disorder, neuroticism, impulsiveness, etc.)	Hedonic versus eudaimonic happiness; virtue ethics and character strengths; self-determination theory; personal expressiveness; psychological well-being; purpose and meaning in life; flourishing; orientations to happiness; resilience; and satisfaction of the full spectrum of human needs	Life satisfaction at the meta-cognitive level mediated by a process involving high personal growth result in high levels of eudaimonia at the developmental level; and conversely, life dissatisfaction mediated by a process involving low personal growth result into low levels of eudaimonia
Positive mental health defined at a social-ecological level = **socio-eudaimonia (eudaimonia + social & moral development)**	Individuals experiencing a preponderance of social resources (social acceptance, social actualization, social contribution, social integration, social harmony, social belongingness, social attachment, familial attachment, etc.) relative to social constraints (social alienation, social discord, social exclusion, ostracism, etc.)	Social well-being, social harmony need to belong, attachment theory; social exclusion and ostracism	High levels of eudaimonia at the developmental level mediated by a process involving high social and moral development result into high levels of socio-eudaimonia at the social-ecological level; and conversely, low levels of eudaimonia mediated by a process involving low social and moral development result into low levels of socio-eudaimonia

research in the social and behavioral sciences. Specifically, he asserts that life satisfaction is an inverse function of the perceived discrepancy between what one has and *what one wants*—the greater the discrepancy the higher the dissatisfaction. This principle is grounded in aspiration theory (e.g., Lewin et al., 1944). The following survey question illustrates this perceived discrepancy: "Consider your life as a whole. How does it measure up to your general aspirations or what you want?" Response categories vary from "not at all" (=1), through "half as well as what you want" (=4) to "matches or is better than what you want" (=7).

Life satisfaction is also hypothesized a direct function of the perceived discrepancy between one has and *what others have*—the greater the discrepancy the higher the dissatisfaction. This principle is grounded by much research in social comparison theory (e.g., Wills, 1981). The following survey question illustrates this perceived discrepancy: "Consider your life as a whole. How does it measure up to the average for most people your own age in this area?" Response categories vary from "far below average" (=1), through "average" (=4) to "far above average" (=7).

Furthermore, life satisfaction is hypothesized a direct function of the perceived discrepancy between one has and *the best one has had in the past*—the greater the discrepancy the higher the dissatisfaction. This principle is grounded by much research in developmental psychology in which children, around the ages of four and five make evaluations based on this standard of comparison compared to older children who make satisfaction judgments using social comparisons with similar others (e.g., Suls & Sanders, 1982). The following survey question illustrates this perceived discrepancy: "Consider your life as a whole. How does it measure up to the best in your previous experience?" Response categories vary from "far below the previous best" (=1), through "matches the previous best" (=4) to "far above the previous best" (=7).

Continuing with the fourth standard of comparison (*what one expected to have 3 years ago*), a similar principle applies. This principle is grounded by much research in quality-of-life studies involving life satisfaction judgments in which the individual compares his current status with the past and noting progress (prompting a satisfaction judgment) or lack of progress (prompting a dissatisfaction judgment) (e.g., Campbell, Converse, & Rodgers, 1976). The following survey question illustrates this perceived discrepancy: "Compared to what you expected to have, does your life offer extremely less (=1), about what you expected (=4), or extremely more (=7)?"

The fifth standard of comparison, *what one expects to have in 5 years*, is what we may call "predictive expectation." Life satisfaction is based on anticipation of meeting future needs. In a survey context, respondents are asked the following: "Consider your life as a whole. How does it measure up to what you expect 5 years from now? Do you expect it to offer extremely less, much more, etc.?"

What one deserves is based on much research in equity theory (e.g., Walster, Berscheid, & Walster, 1976). That is, people feel satisfied with their lives when they feel that they have gotten what they deserve in life. Equity theory asserts that people become satisfied with a specific output given a specific input. For example, an employee may feel dissatisfied with pay when s/he perceives that they deserve more pay because they invested much time and energy, compared to other employee who invested less time and energy with the same pay. The following survey question illustrates this perceived discrepancy: "Consider your life as a whole. How does it measure up to the life you think you deserve?" Response categories vary from "far below what is deserved" (=1), through "matches exactly what is deserved" (=4) to "far above what is deserved" (=7).

Finally, we have the standard of comparison of *what one needs*. People feel dissatisfied with their lives when they perceive that their needs are not met. This principle is supported by much of the research involving person-fit theory (e.g., Caplan, 1983). The following survey question illustrates this perceived discrepancy: "Consider your life as a whole. How does it measure up to the life you think you need?" Response categories vary from "far below what is needed" (=1), through "matches exactly what is needed" (=4) to "far above what is needed" (=7).

A study involving nearly 700 university undergraduates (Michalos, 1985) showed that multiple discrepancies explained 49% of the variance in a happiness measure,[1] 53% in a measure of life satisfaction,[2] and 50% or more in domain satisfaction (7 out of the 12 domain satisfaction ratings). The domains involved in the survey were health, finances, family, job, friendships, housing, area recreation, religion, self-esteem, transportation, and education.

Michalos and colleagues studied a standard of comparison in more depth, namely the *have-relevant others discrepancy*. Here are examples of this research. Michalos (1991) studied the role of the comparison gap between oneself and others among college students and the effect of that gap on life satisfaction and happiness. The social comparison measure was based on asking students how they compared to other students. Michalos found that the social comparison gap was one of the strongest correlates of life satisfaction and happiness. Upward social comparison (comparison of oneself with another who is better off) tends to generate dissatisfaction, whereas downward comparison (comparison of oneself with another who is worse off) generates satisfaction. Similarly, Michalos (1993) found a significant social comparison effect in a variety of life domains. The social comparison effect was a significant predictor of satisfaction with health, religion, education, and recreation in every nation studied. Further evidence comes from data pertaining to income. *Have-relevant others discrepancy* refers to the comparison of one's level of income to the income of others who are significant to the person making the comparison in some ways such as work colleagues and associates (Lance, Mallard, & Michalos, 1995).

Congruity Life Satisfaction

Congruity life satisfaction theory (Meadow, Mentzer, Rahtz, & Sirgy, 1992; Sirgy et al., 1995) is highly akin to multiple discrepancies theory. The central tenet of this theory is that life satisfaction is function of comparison between perceived life accomplishments and a set of standards, namely standards related to derivative sources (accomplishments of relatives, friends, and associates; past accomplishments, average person in a similar occupation, etc.) and different forms (one's view of the ideal life, the deserved life, the minimum tolerable life, etc.). Meadow et al. (1992) report two studies involving the elderly that demonstrated reliability and validity of the measure, Specifically, the measure was found to have construct validity through:

---

[1]The measurement of happiness with life as a whole was based on the following survey item: "Considering your life as a whole, would you describe it as very unhappy (=1), unhappy (=2 or 3), mixed (=4), happy (=5 or 6), or very happy (=7)?"

[2]The measurement of life satisfaction was based on the following survey item: "How do you feel about your life as a whole right now?" Response categories ran from "terrible" (=1), through "mixed dissatisfying and satisfying" (=4) to "delightful" (=7).

- High and positive correlations with the Delighted-Terrible Life Satisfaction Scale;
- Significant correlations (as hypothesized) with cognitive age, income, employment, education, marital status, social contact, activity, religiosity, morale, television viewership, and self-rated health; and
- Nonsignificant correlations (as hypothesized) with chronological age, gender, and parenthood.

In addition, the Sirgy et al. (1995) study reported more construct validity results involving six samples from different countries (USA, Canada, Australia, Turkey, and China). The same construct validity hypotheses, tested in the Meadow et al. (1992) study, were retested in the Sirgy et al. (1995) study and the results were again supportive. The key theoretical tenet is life satisfaction can be captured through a summative (or average) index involving a set of judgments about one's life accomplishments using a set of different standards. To reiterate, the authors argued that referent standards used in the evaluation of life accomplishments may involve a source and a form. The *source of a standard* refers to the principal source of information on which the standard is based. Five sources of standards are identified:

1. *A standard based on the life accomplishments of relatives*: An example of a survey item: "Compared to the ACCOMPLISHMENTS OF YOUR RELATIVES (e.g., parents, brother, sister, etc.), how satisfied are you?" Responses are captured on a 6-point rating scale: from "Very Dissatisfied" or 1 to "Very Satisfied" or 6;
2. *A standard based on the life accomplishments of friends and associates*: An example of a survey item: "Compared to the ACCOMPLISHMENTS OF YOUR FRIENDS AND ASSOCIATES, how satisfied are you?" Responses are captured on a 6-point rating scale: from "Very Dissatisfied" or 1 to "Very Satisfied" or 6;
3. *A standard based on past experience*: An example of a survey item: "Compared to WHERE YOU HAVE BEEN AND HOW FAR YOU HAVE COME ALONG (the progress you have made, the changes you have gone through, or the level of growth you have experienced), how satisfied are you?" Responses are captured on a 6-point rating scale: from "Very Dissatisfied" or 1 to "Very Satisfied" or 6;
4. *A standard based on self-concept or perceived strengths and weaknesses*: An example of a survey item: "Compared to WHAT YOU HAVE EXPECTED FROM YOUR SELF ALL ALONG CONSIDERING YOUR RESOURCES, STRENGTHS, AND WEAKNESSES, how satisfied are you?" Responses are captured on a 6-point rating scale: from "Very Dissatisfied" or 1 to "Very Satisfied" or 6; and
5. *A standard based on the average person in a similar position:* An example of a survey item: "Compared to the ACCOMPLISHMENTS OF MOST PEOPLE IN YOUR POSITION, how satisfied are you?" Responses are captured on a 6-point rating scale: from "Very Dissatisfied" or 1 to "Very Satisfied" or 6.

The *form of a standard* in the evaluation of life accomplishments involve the following standards:

1. *A standard based on ideal outcomes*: An example of a survey item: "Compared to your LIFETIME GOALS, IDEALS, AND WHAT YOU HAD IDEALLY HOPED TO BECOME, how satisfied are you?" Responses are captured on a 6-point rating scale: from "Very Dissatisfied" or 1 to "Very Satisfied" or 6;

2. *A standard based on expected ("should be") outcomes*: An example of a survey item: "Compared to WHAT YOU FEEL YOU SHOULD HAVE ACCOM- PLISHED SO FAR, how satisfied are you?" Responses are captured on a 6-point rating scale: from "Very Dissatisfied" or 1 to "Very Satisfied" or 6;

3. *A standard based on deserved outcomes:* An example of a survey item: "Com- pared to what you feel you DESERVED TO HAVE HAPPENED TO YOU CONSIDERING ALL THAT YOU'VE WORKED FOR, how satisfied are you?" Responses are captured on a 6-point rating scale: from "Very Dissatisfied" or 1 to "Very Satisfied" or 6;

4. *A standard based on minimum tolerable outcomes*: An example of a survey item: "Compared to WHAT YOU FEEL IS THE MINIMUM OF WHAT ANYONE IN YOUR POSITION SHOULD HAVE ACCOMPLISHED (AND BE ABLE TO ACCOMPLISH), how satisfied are you?" Responses are captured on a 6-point rating scale: from "Very Dissatisfied" or 1 to "Very Satisfied" or 6; and

5. *A standard based on predicted outcomes*: An example of a survey item: "Com- pared to WHAT YOU MAY HAVE PREDICTED ABOUT YOURSELF BECOMING, how satisfied are you?" Responses are captured on a 6-point rating scale: from "Very Dissatisfied" or 1 to "Very Satisfied" or 6.

Temporal Satisfaction

Pavot, Diener, and Suh (1998) developed the Temporal Satisfaction with Life Scale (TSWLS). This measure of life satisfaction captures a life satisfaction judgment with different time frames, namely the person's past, present, and future life. The TSWLS was developed based on Diener, Emmons, Larsen, and Griffin (1985) Satisfaction with Life Scale (SWLS); the SWLS captures life satisfaction from the perspective of the present life. The TSWLS consists of 15 items focusing on life satisfaction with a past time frame (e.g., "I am satisfied with my life in the past"), a present time frame (e.g., "I am satisfied with my life"), and a future time frame (e.g., "I will be satisfied with my life in the future"). Survey responses to the TSWLS items are captured on a 4-point Likert-type scale (from 1 = "strongly disagree" to 4 = "strongly agree"). The authors report results demonstrating discriminant validity among these three dimen- sions of life satisfaction. In other words, respondents were able to discriminate between their past, present, and future satisfaction with life. The TSWLS shows good psychometric properties and is widely used in quality-of-life research (e.g. McIntosh, 2001; Murphy, McDevitt-Murphy, & Barnett, 2005).

What is most interesting is the relationship between the TSWLS and measures of eudaimonia. Here is an example of a study demonstrating a positive association between these two constructs. Proyer, Gander, Wyss, and Ruch (2011) conducted a

Table 5.2 Ontological well-being

	Affective evaluations	Cognitive evaluations
Past	Affective reactions to evaluation of one's past circumstances (e.g., feelings of anger with oneself, regret, sadness about the past, feelings of joy)	Recall of salient past events (good and bad); reminiscence and life review
Present	One's emotional reactions to what they are currently doing	Evaluation of life as a whole in current circumstances
Future	Affective reactions such as anxiety, hope, and optimism	One's perception of one's future—optimistic or pessimistic outlook on life

Source: Adapted from Simsek (2009)

study demonstrating how aspects of temporal life satisfaction judgments are related to different character strengths (an important aspect of eudaimonic well-being). An online sample of 1087 women completed the Values in Action Inventory of Strengths and the TSWLS. The results indicate that character strength related to curiosity, hope, gratitude, love, and zest are associated with judgments of present life satisfaction. Appreciation of beauty and excellence as character strengths were associated with judgments of past life satisfaction, more so in older than younger individuals. The results also show that judgments of future life satisfaction are associated with religiousness as a form of character strength. In sum, the study underlines the importance of five key strengths that are associated with judgments of life satisfaction with different temporal frames.

Simsek (2009) has argued that current conceptualizations of subjective well-being focus on unifying the affective (emotional well-being, positive/negative affect, and happiness) and cognitive dimensions (life satisfaction, domain satisfaction, psychological well-being, and eudaimonia), but these attempts have been atheoretical. The author develops a new meta construct called "ontological well-being" that serves to integrate the affective and cognitive dimensions. Ontological well-being is based on the notion that life is a personal project—a goal we desire for its own sake. This personal project can best be viewed from a temporal perspective: past, present, and future. Therefore, the ultimate personal project as life (eudaimonia, personal growth, and psychological well-being) is evaluated cognitively and affectively. The nature of these evaluations is best described in a 2 × 3 matrix below (see Table 5.2).

In the same vein, Durayappah (2011) proposed a 3P model designed to integrate disparate subjective well-being concepts. The 3P model also breaks down subjective well-being along a temporal dimension: past, present, and future. The past component of subjective well-being focuses on happiness that comes from reminiscing, expressions of gratitude, and being able to derive meaning from past experiences. Much of the evidence reflects processes and outcomes related to evaluation of past experiences. Examples of subjective well-being constructs and measures directly related to the "past" include the happiness measure (Fordyce, 1988) and the Satisfaction With Life Scale (Pavot & Diener, 1993). The present component of subjective well-being focuses on positive emotions, flow experiences, and emotional experiences related to self-determination. Much of the evidence reflects processes and outcomes related to the actual experience of a life event. Examples of subjective well-being constructs and measures directly related to the "present" include the PANAS (Watson, Clark, & Tellegen, 1988), experiential sampling (Kahneman, Krueger, Schkade, Schwarz, & Stone, 2004), and the U-Index (Kahneman & Riis, 2005). The future component of subjective well-being focuses on anticipation of happiness, optimism, and issues dealing with life goals. Much of the evidence here reflects processes and outcomes related to expectations and future prospects. Examples of subjective well-being constructs and measures directly related to the "future" include anticipation such as the Savoring Beliefs Inventory (Bryant, 2003), and Orientation of Life Goals Scale (Roberts & Robins, 2000).

Social Comparison

Life satisfaction judgments are also based on social comparisons. That is, people compare themselves with others in relation to life events and outcomes. Such comparison influence feelings of satisfaction or dissatisfaction in life overall. Specifically, *downward comparisons* (comparing one's life circumstance to another person's circumstance that is worse than one's own) tend to generate feelings of satisfaction with life overall, whereas *upwards comparisons* (comparing one's life circumstance to another person's circumstance that is better than one's own) are associated with dissatisfaction. Much research in quality of life suggests that social comparison plays an important role in subjective well-being (see Diener & Fujita, 1996, for a review of the literature). Consider the following example of social comparison studies involving measures of subjective well-being:

- Clark (1996) provided evidence suggesting that unemployment is associated more strongly with lower subjective well-being in regions where unemployment is low than where it is high. This finding signals a social comparison process. That is, people who are unemployed may feel worse when they compare themselves to others and notice that most of these "others" are employed.
- Clark and Oswald (1996) found that job satisfaction is not a function of the absolute level of pay but pay relative to other co-workers with the same education and job classification (cf. Brown, Gardner, Oswald, & Qian, 2003).
- Similarly, in a household survey respondents' satisfaction with their income was found to be dependent on the income generated by other people within the same household. That is, people feel good about their income (and therefore life satisfaction) if they make more money than others in the same household (Neumark & Postlewaite, 1998).
- Luttmer (2005) conducted a large-scale survey in the United States and used social comparison theory to explain his study findings. He found evidence that income of one's neighbor is negatively correlated with one's life satisfaction (the more you observe your neighbor making more money than you the less happy

you feel about your life). In other words, people may feel bad about their lives when they compare themselves to neighbors who make more money than they do (also see Barrington-Leigh & Helliwell, 2008; D'Ambrosio & Frick, 2007; Ferrer-i-Carbonell, 2005; Helliwell & Haung, 2008; Georgellis, Tsitsianis, & Yin, 2009; Stutzer, 2004).

- Diener (2009) discussed social comparison as a possible mediator between income and subjective well-being. People may only know how satisfied they should be (as indicated by their self-reports) by comparing their financial situation with that of others. For example, Morawetz (1977) has provided evidence suggesting that a community with less equal incomes was less happy than a community with more equal income.
- Frieswijk, Buunk, Steverink, and Slaets (2004) examined the effects of social comparison on the life satisfaction of the elderly. The study involved a sample of 455 community-dwelling older people. Sample respondents were exposed to a fictitious interview with either an upward or downward target. The focus topic is about frailty in old age. Those who processed the downward comparison interviews rated their life satisfaction high. In contrast, those who processed the upward comparison interviews reported lower levels of life satisfaction.

Frequency of Positive Affect

Given the fact that life satisfaction judgments are based domain satisfaction and given that domain satisfaction is mostly based on positive and negative affect, it seems reasonable to argue that the frequency of life satisfaction judgments is a construct highly related with the frequency of positive affect. As such, the reader should benefit by becoming familiar with the research on frequency versus intensity of positive affect. Succinctly put, research has shown that frequency of affect is a better indicator of subjective well-being than intensity of affect, given that frequency is more associated with long-term emotional well-being than intensity (Diener, Lucas, & Oishi, 2002). More specifically, Diener et al. (2009) argued that subjective well-being is more strongly associated with the frequency and duration of positive emotions, not with the intensity of those emotions. For instance, individuals who experience high levels of subjective well-being may rarely experience intense feelings such as euphoria. The authors explain this phenomenon as follows: Intense positive feelings often have costs in the form of experiencing intense negative feelings in negative situations, which in turn offset the contribution of intense positive feelings to global feelings of life satisfaction. In other words, happiness is not greatest when one experiences frequent (but mild) positive affect and only minimal amounts of non-intense, negative affect. That is, frequent positive affect is both necessary and sufficient to produce high levels of subjective well-being. Although intense positive experiences may be desirable when they are momentarily experienced, they are not necessarily related to long-term happiness because of the adverse side effects, as well as because of their rarity.

These authors conducted three studies assessing the moods of their subjects over a period of 6–8 weeks and measured both the frequency and intensity of positive affect. This was done by assessing both frequency and intensity at the end of the day measurement times, as well as at random moments throughout each day. Frequency of positive affect was operationalized as the percentage of time subjects were experiencing positive affect at levels exceeding their level of negative affect. Intensity of positive affect was captured as the average intensity of positive affect when the person was experiencing more positive than negative affect (cf. Schimmack & Diener, 1997). The results across the three studies show that the frequency of positive affect was much stronger predictor of several measures of global life satisfaction than positive emotional intensity. Furthermore, these results were found to generalize to nonself-report measures of subjective well-being. Specifically, in one study the authors obtained several nonself-report measures of happiness: an expert rating of well-being based on a structured written interview; peer reports of happiness; and a memory based affect balance measure of well-being comprised of the number of happy versus unhappy life events subjects could recall in a timed period. Each of these well-being measures was predicted by the daily relative frequency and intensity of positive affect of subjects. The results indicated that frequency was a stronger predictor of the nonself-report measures of happiness compared to intensity. In sum, Diener, Sandvik, and Pavot were able to clearly demonstrate that self, peer, and expert ratings, as well as a memory-based assessment of happiness, all seem to be more strongly predicted by frequency of positive affect suggesting that the frequency of positive affect is a key factor in subjective well-being.

Homeostatically Protected Mood

Another stream of research supporting the concept positive balance involves research under the rubric of homeostatically protected mood (HPMood; see Capic, Li, & Cummins, 2018; Cummins, 2010; Cummins et al., 2018). This concept asserts that each individual has a set-point for their normal level of life satisfaction. This set-point is a genetically determined, scoring on 80 points on a 100-point rating scale (varying from low to high life satisfaction). This set-point is not easily modifiable. While life satisfaction is at a constant level, emotions are experienced causing shifts in the set-point. This shift creates an imbalance driving homeostatic forces to restore life satisfaction to its set-point. Thus, affective experience normally oscillates around its set-point. Cummins (2017) argues that given the set-point (around 80 points) to tilt towards the positive pole (100 points), there may be adaptive advantage. This "positive balance" is associated with the benefits of positive emotions such as enhanced friendliness, problem solving, and resource building. However, according to Cummins, this balanced state of positivity also has the downside of ego-centric information processing and an exaggerated sense of control and risk-taking. For example, engaging in a social situation induces positive emotions, which in turn facilitates friendliness. However, doing so reduces the influence of negative emotions, thereby increasing risk-taking. Homeostatic forces would then regulate emotions to restore subjective well-being to the set-point. As such, positive and negative deviations from the set-point are temporally limited. That is not to say that the set-point cannot decrease with repeated negative deviations causing depression (Cummins, 2010).

Given homeostatic imbalance, a set of homeostatic buffers are activated to restore balance. These buffers involve unconscious defenses, behavior, and cognitive defenses. Thus, positive or negative deviations from the set-point tend to activate the buffers to restore homeostasis. These buffers tend to be activated more forcefully in response to negative than to positive deviations to the set-point, because negative affect is associated with survival. Chronic negative deviations from the set-point can overwhelm the buffers resulting in chronic negative homeostatic imbalance (i.e., psychopathological conditions such as depression).

Cummins (2017) argues further that behaviors inducing positive deviations are not that adaptive either. This is because when an experience is pleasurable, people become motivated to prolong the experience. This situation is not considered adaptive because it biases the individual to make unrealistic and impulsive decisions. As such, Cummins argues strong positive emotions are naturally not maintained for long. As such, behaviors reflective of positive experiences tend to wear off quickly allowing the individual to return to his or her set-point. In contrast, behavior reflective of negative experiences do not wear off easily. As a matter of fact, they become consolidated over time. People disengage from behaviors causing negative affect to reduce the probability of encountering future negative experiences. Thus, learning is predicated on negative experiences. People establish life routines that make daily experiences positive, predictable, and manageable. Hence, positive experiences wear off because of habituation, whereas negative experiences are consolidated through learning. For example, people become habituated to winning a big prize (positive experience). While this situation causes positive feelings because the experience is so much more positive than the set-point, it also may cause the set-point to shift upward, which in turn is likely to dampen the experience of positive emotions arising from future positive deviations. However, the opposite occurs in relation to negative experiences. For example, if the individual suffers from the onset of a disease, the negative affect shifts the set-point to a lower level. The individual learns from this experience to help cope with the disease to reduce future negativity.

As such, research under the rubric of the HPMood seems to be consistent with the concept of positive balance—more positivity than negativity. The HPMood concept also supports the notion that life satisfaction judgments are made frequently and biased towards the positive than negative poles of satisfaction. Furthermore, life satisfaction judgments are always made in relation to a referent, and this referent could be explicit or implicit in consciousness. That is, a life satisfaction judgment can be made explicitly with a referent or standard of comparison (e.g., comparing one's satisfaction with current life against satisfaction with past circumstances) or implicitly with a referent that the individual may not be consciously aware of, or what Professor Cummins calls the "set point." One can view Cummins' set point to be a referent capturing life satisfaction of the past.

Emergence

Understanding the construct of domain segmentation is a prerequisite to understanding how domain satisfaction influences the formation of life satisfaction judgments, a topic which I previously addressed in the context of *bottom-up theory of life satisfaction* (Andrews & Withey, 1976; Campbell et al., 1976). See Fig. 5.1.

To reiterate, bottom-up spillover is the spillover of affect from subordinate life domains to superordinate ones, specifically from life domains such as leisure, family,

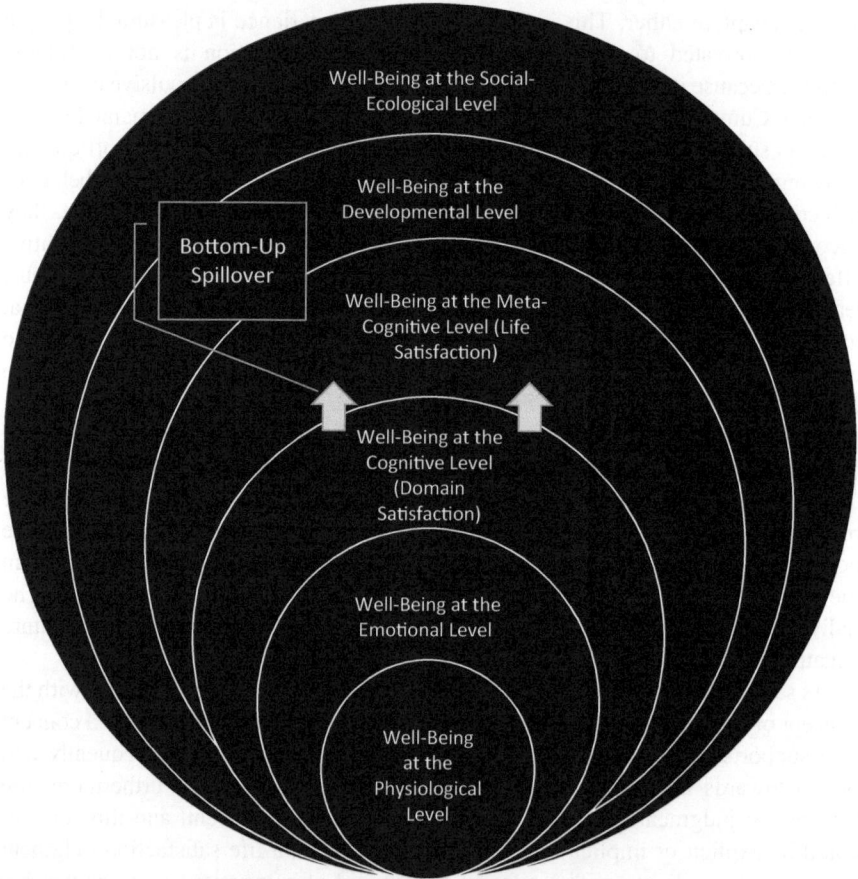

Fig. 5.1 Emergence: well-being at the meta-cognitive level (life satisfaction) influenced by well-being at the cognitive level (domain satisfaction) mediated by a process of bottom-up spillover

job, and health to overall life. That is, feelings within a given life space within the overall hierarchy of life experiences (captured subjectively as cognitions) spill vertically from bottom (most concrete cognitions) to top (most abstract cognitions).

Things happen to people, both positive and negative. They get divorced; they experience death in the family; they find themselves in financial debt; etc. These are examples of negative life events. With respect to positive life events, they may fall in love; they get promoted at work and get a raise; their grown-up children fall in love and get married. And so on! Positive life events, of course, produce positive affect; and conversely, negative life events produce negative affect. Positive and negative affect related to these life events judgments of life satisfaction. There is much evidence suggesting that certain events may cause lasting positive effects (Diener, 2009). For example, evidence shows that plastic surgery may have long-lasting effects on psychological well-being (e.g., Rankin, Borah, Perry, & Wey, 1998). Divorce (Lucas, 2005), unemployment (Lucas, Clark, Georgellis, & Diener, 2003), and the onset of long-term disability (Lucas, 2007) are all related to changes in life satisfaction. Good events are related to positive affect, and bad events are related to negative affect. Domain satisfaction is determined by satisfaction with life events. For example, satisfaction with material life is mostly determined by satisfaction with the monetary value of one's house, car, furniture, clothing, savings, jewelry, accessories, etc. A person's evaluation of these dimensions of the material domain (and/or the direct experience of positive and/or negative affect) can be viewed as satisfaction/dissatisfaction with life events related to material life. Thus, life satisfaction is determined mostly by domain satisfaction. Domain satisfaction is determined mostly by satisfaction with life events related the respective domains.

Figure 5.2 shows the determinants of life satisfaction. Specifically, *life satisfaction* deals with cognitive evaluations of life overall and salient life domains. One's evaluation of one's own life is determined by an aggregation of evaluations of positive and negative events of important life domains (e.g., leisure life, work life, family life, community life, social life, and sex life) or recall of those evaluations made in the past from memory. The evaluation of each life domain is determined by a host of evaluations of life events in that domain or simply one's assessment of positive and negative affect in that domain.

To better appreciate the concepts of domain satisfaction and life satisfaction the reader can benefit from knowing something about how well-being researchers measure these constructs. The Quality of Life Index, developed by Ferrans and Powers (1985), is an example of a measure capturing domain satisfaction. See Table 5.3.

Domain satisfaction ratings are typically treated as independent variables (predictors) whereas life satisfaction is treated as the dependent variable (criterion). See examples of measures the life satisfaction as the dependent variable in the appendix section of my book on *The Psychology of Quality of Life* (Sirgy, 2012) at the end of the book. However, for the sake of convenience here is one example. The European Social Values Survey is nationally representative across 20 European countries. It employs the following item: "All things considered, how satisfied are you with your life as a whole?" The response scale is a 10-point rating scale ranging from "Dissatisfied" to "Satisfied."

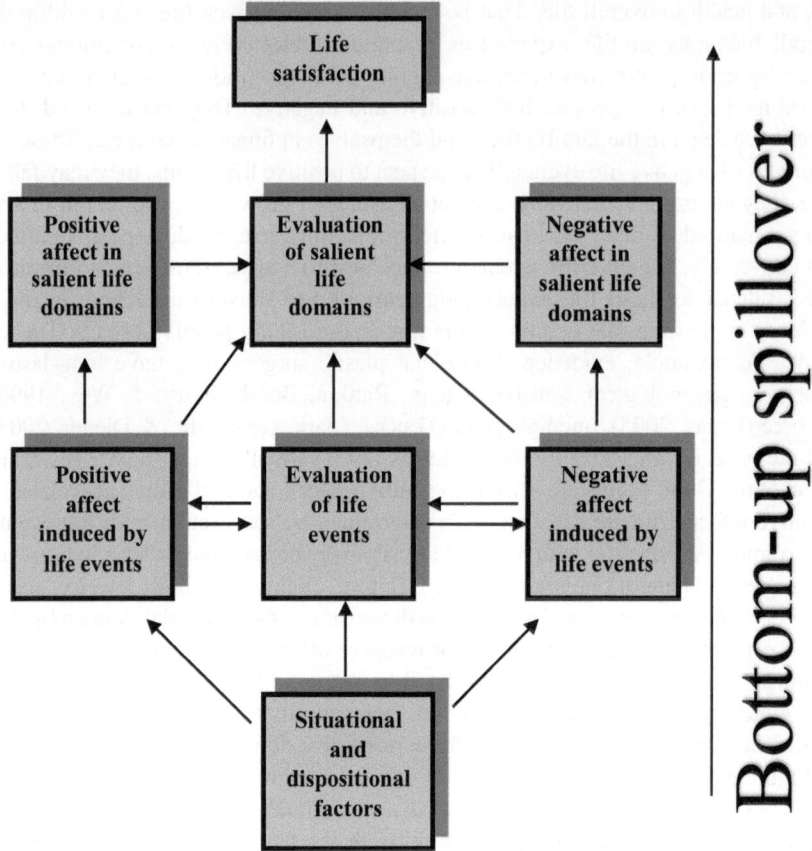

Fig. 5.2 How life satisfaction is determined through a bottom-up process

The concept of bottom-up spillover has been used by well-being researchers to explain the effects of certain domain satisfaction on overall life satisfaction (e.g., Campbell et al., 1976; Chen, Ye, Chen, & Tung, 2010; Diener, 1984; Diener et al., 1999; Efraty, Sirgy, & Siegel, 2000; Gonzalez, Coenders, Saez, & Casas, 2010; Neal, Sirgy, & Uysal, 1999; Sirgy, Hansen, & Littlefield, 1994; Sirgy et al., 1998, Sirgy, Lee, Larsen, & Wright, 1998; Sirgy, Mentzer, Rahtz, & Meadow, 1991; Sirgy, Rahtz, Cicic, & Underwood, 2000; Wu & Yao, 2007). The argument is that life satisfaction can be explained and predicted from domain satisfaction.

Diener (1984), in his classic literature review article that has cited widely, concluded that life satisfaction is mostly determined by domain satisfaction. In commenting on Campbell's (1981) seminal study, he stated the following:

> … the highest correlation was satisfaction with self (.55), suggesting that people must have self-esteem to be satisfied with their lives. Satisfaction with standard of living and with family life were also highly correlated with life satisfaction, whereas the correlation for satisfaction with work was moderate (.37), and satisfaction with health and community were somewhat lower (.29) (Diener, 1984, p. 552).

Table 5.3 The quality-of-life index

This index involves asking respondents to report their degree of satisfaction ("how satisfied are you with?") with the following life domains and experiences
• "Your relationship with your spouse," • "Your friends," • "Your standard of living," • "Your ability to meet non-financial family responsibilities," • "Your usefulness to others," • "Amount of non-job stress or worries in your life," • "Your financial independence," • "Your leisure time activities," • "Your achievement of personal goals," • "Your happiness in general," • "Your health," • "Size of the city in which you live in," • "Your religious life," • "Your family's happiness,"
Responses are recorded on a six-point scale varying from "very dissatisfied" to "very satisfied." the quality-of-life index is computed by average the satisfaction ratings across all life domains

Source: Adapted from Ferrans and Powers (1985)

In sum, the question posed is how domain satisfaction contributes to life satisfaction through an emergence process involving a bottom-up process? The answer is that *domain satisfaction at the cognitive level, mediated by a bottom-up spillover process at the meta-cognitive level, result in life satisfaction; and conversely, domain dissatisfaction mediated by a bottom-up process result in life dissatisfaction.*

Conclusion

A definition of positive mental health based on the concept of positive balance at the meta-cognitive level is offered in this chapter. To reiterate, this definition is as follows: Individuals characterized as having positive mental health tend to experience a preponderance of positive evaluations about one's life using certain standards of comparison (satisfaction with one's life compared to one's past life, the life of family members, etc.) relative to negative evaluations about one's life using similar or other standards of comparison. I then discussed six programs of research supporting this definition of positive balance at the meta-cognitive level: multiple discrepancies theory, congruity life satisfaction, temporal life satisfaction, social comparison, frequency of positive affect, and homeostatically protected mood. Then, I tried to make the case that life satisfaction, the focal well-being construct at the meta-cognitive level, is a psychological phenomenon produced by emergence. Specifically, life satisfaction is determined mostly by domain satisfaction mediated through a bottom-up spillover process.

The next chapter focuses on positive balance as viewed from the developmental level of analysis. I will focus on the concept of eudaimonia and show that life satisfaction (well-being at the meta-cognitive level) plays an important role in the "emergence" of well-being at that developmental level, namely eudaimonia. A definition of positive balance at the developmental level is discussed with supportive evidence from nine programs of research: hedonic versus eudaimonic happiness; virtue ethics and balance; self-determination theory; personal expressiveness; psychological well-being; purpose and meaning in life; authentic happiness and orientations to happiness; flourishing; and satisfaction of the full spectrum of human needs.

References

Andrews, F. M., & Withey, S. B. (1976). *Social indicators of well-being: America's perception of life quality*. New York: Plenum.
Barrington-Leigh, C. P., & Helliwell, J. F. (2008). *Empathy and emulation: Life satisfaction and the urban geography of comparison groups* (NBER Working Paper 14593). National Bureau of Economic Research.
Brown, G. D. A., Gardner, J., Oswald, A., & Qian, J. (2003, June). *Rank dependence in pay satisfaction*. Paper presented at the Brookings/Warwick Conference, Washington, DC.
Bryant, F. B. (2003). Savoring beliefs inventory (SBI): A scale for measuring beliefs about savouring. *Journal of Mental Health, 12*, 175–196.
Campbell, A. (1981). *The sense of well-being in America: Recent patterns and trends*. New York: McGraw-Hill.
Campbell, A., Converse, P. E., & Rodgers, W. L. (1976). *The quality of American life: Perspectives, evaluations, and satisfactions*. New York: Russell Sage Foundation.
Capic, T., Li, N., & Cummins, R. A. (2018). Confirmation of subjective wellbeing set-points: Foundational for subjective social indicators. *Social Indicators Research, 137*, 1–28.
Caplan, R. D. (1983). Person-environment fit: Past, present, and future. In C. L. Cooper (Ed.), *Stress research* (pp. 35–77). New York: Wiley.
Chen, L. H., Ye, Y.-C., Chen, M.-Y., & Tung, I.-W. (2010). Alegria! Flow in leisure and life satisfaction: The mediating role of event satisfaction using data from acrobatics show. *Social Indicators Research, 99*, 301–313.
Clark, A. E. (1996). Job satisfaction in Britain. *British Journal of Industrial Relations, 34*, 189–217.
Clark, A. E., & Oswald, A. J. (1996). Satisfaction and comparison income. *Journal of Public Economics, 61*, 359–381.
Cummins, R. A. (2010). Subjective wellbeing, homeostatically protected mood and depression: A synthesis. *Journal of Happiness Studies, 11*, 1–17.
Cummins, R. A. (2017). Subjective wellbeing homeostasis. In D. S. Dunn (Ed.), *Oxford bibliographies in psychology* (2nd ed.). New York: Oxford University Press.
Cummins, R. A., Capic, T., Fuller-Tyszkiewicz, M., Hutchinson, D., Olsson, C. A., & Richardson, B. (2018). Why self-report variables inter-correlate: The role of homeostatically protected mood. *Journal of Well-Being Assessment, 2*, 93–114.
D'Ambrosio, C., & Frick, J. R. (2007). Income satisfaction and relative deprivation: An empirical link. *Social Indicators Research, 81*, 497–519.
Day, R. L. (1987). Relationship between life satisfaction and consumer satisfaction. In A. C. Samli (Ed.), *Marketing and quality-of-life interface* (pp. 289–311). Westport, CT: Greenwood.
Diener, E. (1984). Subjective well-being. *Psychological Bulletin, 95*, 542–575.
Diener, E. (2009). Subjective well-being. In E. Diener (Ed.), *The science of well-being: The collected works of Ed Diener* (pp. 11–58). Dordrecht: Springer.
Diener, E., & Fujita, F. (1996). Social comparisons and subjective well-being. In B. Buunk & R. Gibbons (Eds.), *Health, coping, and social comparison*. Hillsdale, NJ: Erlbaum.

Diener, E., Emmons, R. A., Larsen, R. J., & Griffin, S. (1985). The satisfaction with life scale. *Journal of Personality Assessment, 49,* 71–75.

Diener, E., Suh, E. M., Lucas, R. E., & Smith, H. L. (1999). Subjective well-being: Three decades of progress. *Psychological Bulletin, 125,* 276–302.

Diener, E., Lucas, R., & Oishi, S. (2002). Subjective well-being: The science of happiness and life satisfaction. In C. R. Snyder & S. J. Lopez (Eds.), *Handbook of positive psychology* (pp. 63–73). New York: Oxford University Press.

Diener, E., Sandvik, E., & Pavot, W. (2009). Happiness is the frequency, not the intensity of positive versus negative affect. In E. Diener (Ed.), *Assessing well-being* (pp. 213–231). Dordrecht: Springer.

Durayappah, A. (2011). The 3P model: A general theory of subjective well-being. *Journal of Happiness Studies, 12,* 681–716.

Efraty, D., Sirgy, M. J., & Siegel, P. (2000). The job/life satisfaction relationship among professional accountants: Psychological determinants and demographic differences. In E. Diener & D. Rahtz (Eds.), *Advances in quality-of-life theory and research* (Vol. 1, pp. 129–157). Dordrecht: Kluwer Academic.

Ferrans, C. E., & Powers, M. J. (1985). Quality of life index: Development and psychometric properties. *Advances in Nursing Science, 8,* 15–24.

Ferrer-i-Carbonell, A. (2005). Income and well-being: An empirical analysis of the comparison income effect. *Journal of Public Economics, 89,* 997–1019.

Fordyce, M. W. (1988). A review of research on happiness measures: A sixty-second index of happiness and mental health. *Social Indicators Research, 20,* 355–381.

Frieswijk, N., Buunk, B. P., Steverink, N., & Slaets, J. P. (2004). The effect of social comparison information on the life satisfaction of frail older persons. *Psychology and Aging, 19,* 183–198.

Georgellis, Y., Tsitsianis, N., & Yin, Y. P. (2009). Personal values as mitigating factors in the link between income and life satisfaction: Evidence from the European social survey. *Social Indicators Research, 91,* 329–344.

Gonzalez, M., Coenders, G., Saez, M., & Casas, F. (2010). Non-linearity, complexity and limited measurement in the relationship between satisfaction with specific life domains and satisfaction with life as a whole. *Journal of Happiness Studies, 11,* 335–352.

Helliwell, J. F., & Haung, H. (2008). How's your government? International evidence linking good government and well-being. *British Journal of Political Science, 38,* 595–619.

Kahneman, D., & Riis, J. (2005). Living and thinking about it: Two perspective on life. In F. A. Huppert, N. Baylis, & B. Keverne (Eds.), *The science of well-being* (pp. 285–304). Oxford, UK: Oxford University Press.

Kahneman, D., Krueger, A. B., Schkade, D., Schwarz, N., & Stone, A. A. (2004). Toward national well-being accounts. *American Economic Review, 94,* 427–440.

Lance, C. E., Mallard, A. G. C., & Michalos, A. C. (1995). Tests of causal directions of global-life facet satisfaction relationships. *Social Indicators Research, 34,* 69–92.

Lewin, K., et al. (1944). Level of aspiration. In J. M. V. Hunt (Ed.), *Personality and behavior disorders* (pp. 333–378). New York: Ronald Press.

Lucas, R. E. (2005). Time does not heal all wounds: A longitudinal study of reaction and adaptation to divorce. *Psychological Science, 16,* 945–950.

Lucas, R. E. (2007). Long-term disability has lasting effects of subjective well-being: Evidence from two nationally-representative panel studies. *Journal of Personality and Social Psychology, 92,* 717–730.

Lucas, R. E., Clark, A. E., Georgellis, Y., & Diener, E. (2003). Reexamining adaptation and the set-point model of happiness: Reactions to changes in marital status. *Journal of Personality and Social Psychology, 84,* 527–539.

Luttmer, E. F. P. (2005). Neighbours as negatives: Relative earnings and well-being. *Quarterly Journal of Economics, 120,* 963–1002.

McIntosh, C. N. (2001). Report on the construct validity of the temporal satisfaction with life scale. *Social Indicators Research, 54,* 37–56.

Meadow, H. L., Mentzer, J. J., Rahtz, D. R., & Sirgy, M. J. (1992). A life satisfaction measure based on judgment theory. *Social Indicators Research, 26*, 23–59.

Michalos, A. C. (1985). Multiple discrepancies theory (MDT). *Social Indicators Research, 16*, 347–413.

Michalos, A. C. (1986). An application of multiple discrepancies theory (MDT) to seniors. *Social Indicators Research, 18*, 349–373.

Michalos, A. C. (1991). *Global on student well-being. Volume 1: Life satisfaction and happiness.* New York: Springer.

Michalos, A. C. (1993). *Global report on student well-being. Volume IV: Religion, education, recreation, and health.* New York: Springer.

Michalos, A. C., Hatch, P. M., Hemingway, D., Lavallee, L., Hogan, A., & Christensen, B. (2007). Health and quality of life of older people, a replication after six years. *Social Indicators Research, 84*, 127–158.

Morawetz, D. (1977). Income distribution and self-rated happiness: Some empirical evidence. *The Economic Journal, 87*, 511–522.

Murphy, J. G., McDevitt-Murphy, M. E., & Barnett, N. P. (2005). Drink and be merry? Gender, life satisfaction, and alcohol consumption among college students. *Psychology of Addictive Behaviors, 19*, 184–191.

Neal, J., Sirgy, M. J., & Uysal, M. (1999). The role of satisfaction with leisure travel/tourism services and experiences in satisfaction with leisure life and overall life. *Journal of Business Research, 44*, 153–163.

Neumark, D., & Postlewaite, A. (1998). Relative income concerns and the rise in married women's employment. *Journal of Public Economics, 70*, 157–183.

Pavot, W., & Diener, E. (1993). Review of the satisfaction with life scale. *Psychological Assessment, 5*, 164–172.

Pavot, W., Diener, E., & Suh, E. (1998). The temporal satisfaction with life scale. *Journal of Personality Assessment, 70*, 340–354.

Proyer, R. T., Gander, F., Wyss, T., & Ruch, W. (2011). The relation of character strengths to past, present, and future life satisfaction among German-speaking women. *Applied Psychology: Health and Well-Being, 3*(3), 370–384.

Rankin, M., Borah, G. L., Perry, A. W., & Wey, P. D. (1998). Quality-of-life outcomes after cosmetic surgery. *Plastic and Reconstructive Surgery, 102*, 2139–2145.

Roberts, B. W., & Robins, R. W. (2000). Broad dispositions, broad aspirations: The intersection of the big five dimensions and major life goals. *Personal and Social Psychology Bulletin, 26*, 1284–1296.

Schimmack, U., & Diener, E. (1997). Affect intensity: Separating intensity and frequency in repeatedly measured affect. *Journal of Personality and Social Psychology, 73*(6), 1313–1329.

Simsek, O. F. (2009). Happiness revisited: Ontological well-being as a theory-based construct of subjective well-being. *Journal of Happiness Studies, 10*, 505–522.

Sirgy, M. J. (2012). *The psychology of quality of life: Hedonic well-being, life satisfaction, and eudaimonia.* Dordrecht: Springer.

Sirgy, M. J., Mentzer, J. T., Rahtz, D., & Meadow, H. L. (1991). Satisfaction with healthcare marketing services consumption and life satisfaction among the elderly. *Journal of Macromarketing, 11*, 24–39.

Sirgy, M. J., Hansen, D. E., & Littlefield, J. E. (1994). Does hospital satisfaction affect life satisfaction? *Journal of Macromarketing, 14*, 36–46.

Sirgy, M. J., Cole, D., Kosenko, R., Meadow, H. L., Rahtz, R. D., Cicic, M., et al. (1995). Judgment-type life satisfaction measure: Further validation. *Social Indicators Research, 34*, 237–259.

Sirgy, M. J., Lee, D.-J., Kosenko, R., Meadow, H. L., Rahtz, D., Cicic, M., et al. (1998). Does television viewership play a role in the perception of quality of life? *Journal of Advertising, 27*, 125–142.

Sirgy, M. J., Lee, D.-J., Larsen, V., & Wright, N. (1998). Satisfaction with material possessions and general well-being: The role of materialism. *Journal of Consumer Satisfaction/Dissatisfaction and Complaining Behavior, 11*, 103–118.

Sirgy, M. J., Rahtz, D. R., Cicic, M., & Underwood, R. (2000). A method for assessing residents' satisfaction with community-based services: A quality-of-life perspective. *Social Indicators Research, 49*, 279–316.

Stutzer, A. (2004). The role of income aspirations in individual happiness. *Journal of Economic Behavior and Organization, 54*, 89–109.

Suls, J., & Sanders, G. S. (1982). Self-evaluations through social comparison: A developmental analysis. *Review of Personality and Social Psychology, 3*, 171–197.

Walster, E., Berscheid, E., & Walster, G. W. (1976). New directions in equity research. In L. Berkowitz & E. Walster (Eds.), *Advances in experimental social psychology* (pp. 1–42). New York: Academic.

Watson, D., Clark, L. A., & Tellegen, A. (1988). Development and validation of brief measures of positive and negative affect: The PANAS scales. *Journal of Personality and Social Psychology, 54*, 1063–1070.

Wills, T. A. (1981). Doward comparison principles in social psychology. *Psychological Bulletin, 90*(2), 245–262.

Wu, C.-H., & Yao, G. (2007). Importance has been considered in satisfaction evaluation: An experimental examination of Locke's range-of-affect hypothesis. *Social Indicators Research, 81*, 521–541.

Chapter 6
Positive Balance at the Developmental Level: Eudaimonia

Introduction

> . . .it pointed to an alternative approach, a 'negative path' to happiness, that entailed taking a radically different stance towards those things that most of us spend our lives trying to avoid. It involved learning to enjoy uncertainty, embracing insecurity, stopping trying to think positively, becoming familiar with failure, even learning to value death. In short, all these people seemed to agree that in order to be truly happy, we might actually need to be willing to experience more negative emotions—or, at the very least to learn to stop running quite so hard from them.—Oliver Burkeman, The Antidote: Happiness for People Who Can't Stand Positive Thinking (https://www.goodreads.com/quotes/tag/eudaimonia)

Daniel Haybron (2000) makes the distinction among three philosophical concepts of happiness: psychological happiness, prudential happiness, and perfectionist happiness. According to Haybron (2000), *psychological happiness* is indeed a state of mind involving feelings of joy, serenity, and affection. Psychological happiness is the experience of positive emotions over time. *Prudential happiness*, on the other hand, refers to a state of well-being. Psychological happiness may be a necessary but not sufficient condition of prudential happiness. Prudential happiness is achieved when a person achieves a high state of well-being, both mentally and physically. Haybron illustrates this condition by describing a brain in a vat. The brain in a vat may experience perfect bliss (psychological happiness), but physically it is not leading a good life as a person in his or her full humanity (prudential happiness). In other words, happiness is more than feelings of joy. It necessitates engagement in life to realize one's potential. It is what people do in life to achieve personal fulfilment. It is leading the good life. In contrast, *perfectionist happiness* refers to a life that is good in all respects, including a *moral* life. It is a life that is desirable without qualification, both enviable and admirable. Perfectionist happiness is achieved when a person achieves a state of well-being plus leading a moral life. Haybron illustrates the concept of perfectionist happiness by describing an evil person. This person may be experiencing feelings of joy and happiness (high on psychological happiness), is well off in every way (high on prudential happiness) but

M. J. Sirgy, *Positive Balance*, Social Indicators Research Series 80,
https://doi.org/10.1007/978-3-030-40289-1_6

is a parasite to society (low on perfectionist happiness). Perfectionist happiness is what philosophers mean by eudaimonia or eudaimonic well-being.

Ed Diener, the dean of subjective well-being research, has long viewed subjective well-being as an umbrella concept that involves several dimensions: positive/negative affect, domain satisfaction, and judgments of life satisfaction, as well as absence of ill-being (e.g., depression and other forms of psychopathology). Diener and colleagues have long recognized that subjective well-being and eudaimonia, although highly interrelated, are distinct from each other (e.g., Kesebir & Diener, 2009). Consider the following quotation:

> It is important for the purposes of this discussion to emphasize that most of the empirical studies conducted in psychology regarding happiness … conceive of happiness not in the eudaimoinc sense—embodying a value judgment about whether the person is leading a commendable life—but rather in the sense of subjective well-being. Clearly, high subjective well-being and eudaimonic happiness are not necessarily interchangeable concepts, and it is easily imaginable that a person could feel subjectively happy without leading a virtuous life. However, we believe, and many contemporary philosophers … agree, that subjective well-being and eudaimonic well-being are sufficiently close. It is reasonable to use subjective well-being as a proxy for well-being, even if it is not a perfect match. Admittedly, current empirical psychological research cannot directly answer the ancient philosophical question of how to live well. As researchers of subjective well-being, our hope is that we answer this question indirectly by illuminating a *sine qua non* of the good life—namely, subjective well-being (Kesebir & Diener, 2009; p. 62).

Table 6.1 captures a synopsis of much of the discussion in this chapter in the context of the entire book. See the shaded area in the table concerning eudaimonia. Based on the preceding discussion, I offer a definition of positive mental health based on the concept of positive balance at the developmental level. The definition is as follows: *Individuals experiencing a preponderance of positive psychological traits (personal growth, purpose in life, environmental mastery, autonomy, positive relations with others, etc.) relative to negative psychological traits (pessimism, hopelessness, depressive disorder, neuroticism, impulsiveness, etc.).* In the following sections, I discuss nine programs of research supporting this definition of positive balance at the developmental level. These research programs are hedonic versus eudaimonic happiness; virtue ethics and balance; self-determination theory; personal expressiveness; psychological well-being; purpose and meaning in life; authentic happiness and orientations to happiness; flourishing; orientations to happiness, resilience; and satisfaction of the full spectrum of human needs. After describing these programs of research in support of my definition, I'll describe how positive balance expressed in eudaimonia contributes to socio-eudaimonia through emergence.

Table 6.1 Positive mental health defined at various hierarchical levels as positive balance with emergence and focus on the developmental level

Level of analysis	Positive balance as positive mental health	Programs of research	Emergence
Positive mental health defined at a physiological level = **positive and negative neurotransmitters**	Individuals experiencing a preponderance of neurochemicals related to positive emotions (dopamine, serotonin, oxytocin) relative to neurochemicals related to negative emotions (cortisol)	Stress response system); neurobiology of happiness)	
Positive mental health defined at an emotional level = **positive/negative affect or hedonic well-being (positive/negative neurotransmitters + cognitive appraisals)**	Individuals experiencing a preponderance of positive emotions (happiness, joy, serenity, contentment, etc.) relative to negative emotions (anger, sadness, jealousy, envy, depression, etc.)	Positive versus negative affect; broaden and build theory; flow	Positive neurochemicals (dopamine, serotonin, and oxytocin) at the physiological level mediated by a process of cognitive appraisal (positive frame) result into positive affect (happiness, joy, contentment, etc.) at the emotional level; and conversely, negative neurochemicals (cortisol) mediated by a process of cognitive appraisal (negative frame) result into negative affect (anger, sadness, jealousy, envy, depression, etc.)
Positive mental health defined at a cognitive level = **domain satisfaction (positive/negative affect + domain segmentation)**	Individuals experiencing a preponderance of domain satisfaction (satisfaction in salient and multiple life domains such as family life, work life, social life, etc.) relative to dissatisfaction in other life domains	Principle of satisfaction limits; principle of the full spectrum of human developmental needs; principle of diminishing satisfaction	Positive affect (happiness, joy, contentment, etc.) at the emotional level mediated by a process of domain segmentation result into domain satisfaction (satisfied with work life, social life, family life, etc.); and conversely, negative affect (anger, sadness, jealousy, envy, depression, etc.) mediated by a process of domain segmentation result into domain dissatisfaction (dissatisfied with work life, social life, family life, etc.)
Positive mental health defined at a meta-cognitive level = **life satisfaction (domain satisfaction + bottom-up process)**	Individuals experiencing a preponderance of positive evaluations about one's life using certain standards of comparison (satisfaction with one's life compared to one's past life, the life of family members, the life of associates at work, the life of others in the same social circles, etc.) relative to negative evaluations about one's life using similar or other standards of comparison	Multiple discrepancies theory; congruity life satisfaction; temporal life satisfaction; social comparison; frequency of positive affect; homeostatically protected mood	Domain satisfaction (satisfied with work life, social life, family life, etc.) at the cognitive level mediated by a bottom-up process at the meta-cognitive level result in life satisfaction; and conversely. domain dissatisfaction (dissatisfied with work life, social life, family life, etc.) mediated by a bottom-up process result in life dissatisfaction

(continued)

Table 6.1 (continued)

Positive mental health defined at a developmental level = **eudaimonia (life satisfaction + personal growth)**	Individuals experiencing a preponderance of positive psychological traits (self-acceptance, personal growth, purpose in life, environmental mastery, autonomy, positive relations with others, etc.) relative to negative psychological traits (pessimism, hopelessness, depressive disorder, neuroticism, impulsiveness, etc.)	Hedonic versus eudaimonic happiness; virtue ethics and character strengths; self-determination theory; personal expressiveness; psychological well-being; purpose and meaning in life; flourishing; orientations to happiness; resilience; and satisfaction of the full spectrum of human needs	Life satisfaction at the meta-cognitive level mediated by a process involving high personal growth result in high levels of eudaimonia at the developmental level; and conversely, life dissatisfaction mediated by a process involving low personal growth result into low levels of eudaimonia
Positive mental health defined at a social-ecological level = **socio-eudaimonia (eudaimonia + social & moral development)**	Individuals experiencing a preponderance of social resources (social acceptance, social actualization, social contribution, social integration, social harmony, social belonginess, social attachment, familial attachment, etc.) relative to social constraints (social alienation, social discord, social exclusion, ostracism, etc.)	Social well-being, social harmony need to belong, attachment theory; social exclusion and ostracism	High levels of eudaimonia at the developmental level mediated by a process involving high social and moral development result into high levels of socio-eudaimonia at the social-ecological level; and conversely, low levels of eudaimonia mediated by a process involving low social and moral development result into low levels of socio-eudaimonia

Programs of Research Supporting the Definition of Positive Balance

In the next sections I discuss several programs of research supporting my definition of positive balance at the developmental level. These are: hedonic versus eudaimonic happiness, virtue ethics and character strengths, self-determination theory, personal expressiveness, psychological well-being, purpose and meaning in life, flourishing, orientations to happiness, resilience, and satisfaction of the full spectrum of human needs.

Hedonic Versus Eudaimonic Happiness

Well-being researchers have conducted much research distinguishing hedonic from eudaimonic well-being (e.g., Deci & Ryan, 2008; Delle Fave, Brdar, Freire, Vella-Brodrick, & Wissing, 2011; Duckworth & Gross, 2014; Joshanloo, 2016; Munoz

Sastre, 1998; Ryan & Deci, 2000; Ryan, Huta, & Deci, 2008; Schwartz, 2015; Schwartz & Wrzesniewski, 2016; Vitterso, 2016; Waterman, 1993). The hedonic conception of well-being treats well-being in terms of life satisfaction, domain satisfaction, the preponderance of positive over negative affect, as well as the absence of feelings of depression. As such the hedonic view of happiness is equivalent to the traditional conception of subjective well-being as defined by Diener and his colleagues (Diener, 1984; Diener, Suh, Lucas, & Smith, 1999). In contrast, the eudaimonic conception of well-being treats well-being in terms of personal growth and development—cognitive, emotional, social, and moral growth. As such, it is viewed as the cornerstone of positive mental health.

Consider the research by Vitterso, Soholt, Hetland, Alekseeva Thoresen, and Roysamb (2010). They explicitly addressed the theoretical distinction between *hedonic well-being* and *eudaimonic well-being*. They argue that the cybernetic principles underlying hedonic well-being are different from eudaimonic well-being. Goal attainment in the context of hedonic well-being reflects homeostatic balance (i.e., a state of equilibrium and assimilation), which reflects a state of happiness. In contrast, lack of goal attainment reflects a state of disequilibrium that induces feelings of interest, curiosity, challenge, and task absorption. The latter may be reflective of eudaimonic well-being. They conducted several studies demonstrating that the experience of hedonic versus eudaimonic well-being is dependent of the extent to which the task at hand is easy or difficult. The individual is most likely to experience hedonic well-being when the task is easy but eudaimonic well-being when the task is difficult.

Along a similar line of reasoning, Huppert (2009) asserts that eudaimonia is about lives going well. This means that eudaimonia combines the traditional notion of subjective well-being with *effective functioning*. Subjective well-being may focus too much on positive emotions. In contrast, eudaimonia focuses on sustainable well-being in the sense that negative emotions can play a significant and positive role in long-term well-being. People must learn to manage negative emotions to enhance long-term positive emotions. Of course, eudaimonia is undermined when negative emotions are experienced frequently without the benefit of learning and long-term positive emotions. Researchers embracing the concept of eudaimonia view positive emotions more broadly than happiness and contentment. Positive emotions may include interest, engagement, confidence, and affection. Most importantly is the concept of *functioning*, which involves the development of one's potential, having control over life's circumstances, believing that life has meaning, having a purposeful role to play in life, as well as having positive relationships with others.

This research underscores the notion that well-being, construed from the perspective of eudaimonia, should capture elements beyond positive and negative affect, domain satisfaction, and life satisfaction. Well-being, in this context, is a higher-order construct capturing dispositional elements related to happiness, positive personal characteristics and traits that help the individual function in daily life. To function effectively the person must experience not only a certain degree of life satisfaction but also possess certain psychological traits that serve to enhance functioning. Examples of these psychological traits may include environmental mastery and autonomy. By the same token, the individual must not possess psychological traits that are well-known to hinder functioning. Examples of these negative traits include pessimism, hopelessness, depressive disorder, neuroticism, and impulsiveness.

Based on the research distinguishing hedonic well-being from eudaimonia, I believe that the program of research on this topic provides support for a definition of well-being and positive mental health that reflects the notion of positive balance at the developmental level—well-being, as eudaimonia, reflects as state in which the individual experiences a preponderance of positive psychological traits (environmental mastery, autonomy, positive relations with others, etc.) relative to negative psychological traits (pessimism, hopelessness, depressive disorder, neuroticism, impulsiveness, etc.).

Virtue Ethics and Character Strengths

The famous and most renowned Greek philosophers, Plato, Socrates, and Aristotle, associated happiness with *virtue* (e.g., Aristotle, 340 BC/1986; Plato, 360 BC/1892). For example, in Plato's dialogue "Gorgias," Socrates tells Polus, "The men and women who are gentle and good are also happy, as I maintain, and the unjust and evil are miserable" (Plato, 360 BC/1892 translated, p. 529). They believed that people become happy through wisdom and choosing wisely. People do not act irresponsibly towards themselves or others when they choose wisely.

Aristotle, in *Nichomachean Ethics*, written in 350 B.C., provided guidance about how to live a good life, an ethical life (Rowe & Broadie, 2002). Happiness is not necessarily about pleasure. It is about virtue, and virtue is essentially life balance—balance applied to many areas of living. For example, balance in material life is balance between material excess and material deficiency. Too much honor leads to vanity and too little turns to undue humility. Too much amusement becomes buffoonery, too little is dullness. The principle of balance as virtue is to choose deliberate action that avoids both excess and deficiency. Virtue also involves activities that have significant life purpose. This discussion may lead us to postulate that subjective well-being is about living a virtuous life. In turn, living a virtuous life entails balance between polar extremes in the pursuit of life goals. However, one can argue that happiness, in the context of this philosophical discourse, is not simply balance between two polar sets of values but positive balance. That is, balance with more weight given to the positive polar extreme than the negative one.

A related program of research in positive psychology related to virtues is character strengths. Peterson and Seligman (2004) developed a compendium of human virtues, referred to as *Character Strengths and Virtues: A Handbook and Classification*. This "manual" is viewed as the antonym of the *Diagnostic and Statistical Manual*'s list of what is wrong about human beings in terms of mental illness. Related to this manual is the character strength survey by the VIA Institute on Character (viacharacter.org) that allows site visitors to learn about their strengths for the purpose of using their strengths in new and different ways and to further develop them. The authors classified character strengths and virtues into 24 categories organized into six types. The six virtues followed by their 24-character strengths are:

1. *Wisdom and Knowledge*: creativity, curiosity, open-mindedness, love of learning, perspective, innovation
2. *Courage*: bravery, persistence, integrity, vitality, zest
3. *Humanity*: love, kindness, social intelligence
4. *Justice*: citizenship, fairness, leadership
5. *Temperance*: forgiveness and mercy, humility, prudence, self-control
6. *Transcendence*: appreciation of beauty and excellence, gratitude, hope, humor, spirituality.

This manual and the accompanying survey have changed how character strength is understood and used by many to activate positive experiences (e.g., Park & Peterson, 2009; Peterson, Ruch, Beermann, Park, & Seligman, 2007; Niemiec, 2013). The work helped to further promote positive psychotherapy.[1] For example, Flückiger and Grosse Holtforth (2008) have used resource priming to focus on the client's character strengths at the beginning of each therapy session. Character strengths priming leads to resource activation whereby the client interprets his own behavior in a positive light, which facilitates the on-going dynamics in the session leading to enhanced well-being. Character strengths priming was also shown to foster a stronger therapist-client bond across the 20 sessions.

What is the supportive evidence that a character strengths intervention is effective? Quinlan, Swain, and Vella-Brodick (2012) conducted a review of the literature and found small but statistically significant effects of character strength interventions on well-being across eight studies. An example of a study that provided evidence for the effectiveness of a character strengths intervention is Seligman, Rashid, and Parks (2006). Forty mild-to-moderately depressed college students were assigned to two groups: a treatment group and a non-treatment group. Participants in the treatment condition were seen for six weekly two-hour sessions. Each session involved a discussion of the exercise assigned from the previous week and an introduction to a new exercise. Participants carried out their homework assignments and reported back each week on their progress. During the first week, participants were instructed to complete the Values in Action (VIA) Inventory of Character Strengths (Peterson & Seligman, 2004) and use their top five strengths more often in their daily activities. During the second week, participants documented three good things that had happened and explained why these things had occurred. During the third week participants were instructed to write a brief essay on what they wanted to be remembered for the most—a biography of having lived a good life. The following session involved writing a letter of gratitude to someone they may never have had the chance to thank properly, and then reading that letter to the person, personally or by phone.

---

[1]Interested readers are referred to the thought-provoking article on how character strengths can be used to assess and understand the etiology and treatment of psychopathology (Seligman 2015).

During the fifth session, participants were instructed to respond positively and enthusiastically each day to good news received by someone else. The final session involved savoring—taking pleasure in the daily events they normally did not take the time to enjoy. They were instructed to document their feelings related to savoring.[2] As expected, the participants in the treatment group did better than the non-treatment group on self-reports of depression and life satisfaction, and these gains were maintained with no other intervention by the researchers throughout a one-year follow-up, while the baseline levels of depression for the non-treatment group remained unchanged.

The discussion related to character strengths helps establish an argument that well-being and positive mental health involves a preponderance of positive psychological traits (e.g., character strengths) over negative ones (e.g., character weaknesses). Character strengths may include wisdom, knowledge, courage, humanity, justice, temperance, and transcendence. Character weaknesses may include traits such as impulsiveness, dogmatism and close-mindedness, and narcissism. Such a view supports the positive balance view of well-being and positive mental health at the developmental level.

Self-Determination Theory

Self-determination theory (SDT) is attributed to Richard M. Ryan and Edward L. Deci. See their article in the *American Psychologist* summarizing much of the well-being research guided by SDT (Ryan & Deci, 2000). SDT posits that well-being can be enhanced by satisfying three major needs: *competence*, *autonomy*, and *relatedness* (cf. Demir, Ozen, Dogan, Bilyk, & Tyrell, 2011; Howell, Chenot, Hill, & Howell, 2011). These three needs, based on SDT, are essential for personal growth and well-being.

Cognitive evaluation theory (CET) is a precursor of SDT, developed by Deci and Ryan (1985). CET is a sub theory of SDT focusing only on the needs of competence and autonomy. The essence of CET is the notion that there are social and environmental factors (e.g., feedback, communication, rewards) facilitating and undermining intrinsic motivation. In other words, feedback that promotes effectance and freedom from demeaning evaluations can go a long way to enhance intrinsic motivation and well-being. Specifically, feelings of competence conjoin with the sense of autonomy to induce the expression of intrinsic motivation. Intrinsic motivation is operationalized when a person engages an activity (a job activity) because the person is interested in the activity itself instead of the tangential rewards or punishment associated with the activity (e.g., doing the job to earn a living or to avoid the boss' possible reprimand).

---

[2]A version of the material in this section has been discussed in a blog written by the author: https://psychcentral.com/blog/archives/2013/01/27/moving-from-whats-wrong-to-whats-strong-introducing-positive-psychotherapy-ppt/

SDT builds on CET by adding relatedness needs to the list of intrinsic motives that play a major role in well-being. Intrinsic motivation manifests itself through internalization and integration. Self-determination can be viewed along a continuum from "nonself-determined" to "self-determined." When people engage in activities in non-self-determined ways, they are said to be "amotivated." Their behavior is regulated by extrinsic rewards and punishment. They do not sense control over the activity situation (i.e., the perceived locus of causality is impersonal). Therefore, the behavior related to that activity is essentially non-intentional and non-valuing. They do not feel a sense of competence or control engaging that task. The other extreme is self-determined behavior that reflects intrinsic motivation. Intrinsically motivated behavior is inherently internally regulated. People's perception of causality is internal, and their behavior comes across as interested in the activity, that they enjoy the activity and feel quite satisfied. External regulation is behavior directed by external reward and punishment contingencies. Introjected regulation is a relatively controlled form of regulation guided by ego-enhancing feelings such as pride and ego-defensive feelings such as guilt and anxiety. In contrast, regulation through identification involves action guided by feelings of identification. People begin to identify themselves with the activity. Integrated regulation is an advanced form of regulation through identification in which they incorporate the activity fully into the self (i.e., they describe part of their identity in terms of the activity).

The relative internalization of an activity is a function of relatedness, competence, and autonomy. That is, for an activity to be fully internalized, the person must have support from significant others who are either role models or provide moral support, thus satisfying the need for relatedness. The activity must generate feelings of effectance, making the individual feel competent in this endeavor, thus satisfying the need for competence. Furthermore, the individual must make an autonomous decision to engage in the activity. Doing so allows the individual to feel a sense of ownership of the activity, thus satisfying the need for autonomy.

Now let us turn to extrinsic motivation and address psychological traits that may be related to extrinsic motivation. There is a program of research in materialism grounded in self-determination theory demonstrating that materialism is indeed an individual difference variable associated with negative expressions of well-being (Kasser, 2016). Specifically, materialism reflects a set of values and life goals focused on wealth, possessions, image, and status. These values and life goals conflict with values and life goals related to personal growth and the well-being of others. Kasser documented much evidence (correlational as well as experimental) showing that materialistic people

- consume more status products (i.e., buy and consume more status goods and services),
- incur more debt (i.e., have high credit card debt and other loans),
- have little social capital (i.e., poor interpersonal relationships),
- are less environmental responsible (i.e., act in more ecologically destructive ways),
- are less motivated to work and attain higher levels of education, and
- report lower levels of personal and physical well-being.

Furthermore, Kasser reports on successful interventions that encourage intrinsic (or self-transcendent) values and lifegoals and block materialistic messages from the environment.

The point of this discussion is to highlight the notion that personal growth, a focal aspect of eudaimonia, is partly based on intrinsic motivation. The individual experiences personal growth mostly through expressions of intrinsic, not extrinsic motivation. Expressions of intrinsic motivation are reflected in autonomy, competence, and relatedness. As such, one can argue that eudaimonia may involve a preponderance of manifestations of intrinsic motivation (expressions related to autonomy, competence, and relatedness) relative to manifestations of extrinsic motivation. Self-determination research supports the definition of positive balance at the developmental level. That is, well-being and positive mental health at the developmental level involve a preponderance of positive psychological traits related to intrinsic motivation (autonomy, competence, positive relations with others, etc.) relative to negative psychological traits related to extrinsic motivation (materialism, etc.).

Personal Expressiveness

Waterman (1990, 1992, 1993, 2004, 2005; Waterman et al. 2003; Waterman, Schwartz, & Conti, 2008) has long argued that identity development proceeds most successfully when people identify their best potentials and engage in activities that move them toward realizing those potentials. Engagement in those eudaimonistic activities produces feelings of personal expressiveness. These personal expressive feelings, in turn, reinforce the motivation that people feel to continue to engage in those activities. For example, a person may train for a marathon not only because he or she views running as serving instrumental goals such as health or glory but primarily for intrinsic experiential rewards—it makes the person "feel alive" and "feel intensely involved." In other words, engaging in the activity leads the person toward a state of eudaimonia. The key point, though, is that the reward is intrinsic because the intrinsic feelings experienced are an end goal.

Personal expressiveness theory distinguishes two types of activities—those leading to hedonic enjoyment alone and those leading also to personal expressiveness. Activities associated simultaneously with hedonic enjoyment and personal expressiveness are most likely to be pursued in a sustained manner, contributing to self-realization. For example, a woman may enjoy a bicycle run and eating a fine healthy dinner with friends from the bicycling sport club. Both activities are hedonically enjoyable. However, the bicycle exercise is not only hedonically enjoyable but also personally expressive. Bicycle exercise is more likely to involve a rigorous physical activity that serves to actualize the woman's potential to master this sport, whereas having that a fine dinner with friends is likely to be only hedonically satisfying. Waterman and colleagues call activities both hedonically satisfying and personally expressive as "intrinsic motivating activities," whereas activities that are only hedonically satisfying as "hedonic motivating activities." Examples of measurement items capturing hedonic enjoyment include: "When I engage in this activity, I feel more satisfied than I do when I engage in most other activities"; "This activity gives me my strongest sense of enjoyment." Items capturing personal expressiveness include: "This activity gives me the greatest feeling of really being alive"; "When I engage in this activity, I feel more intensely involved than I do when engaged in most other activities." Empirical evidence has demonstrated that these two constructs are highly interrelated. However, there is an asymmetry between the two constructs in the sense that there is a significantly higher percentage of activities high on eudaimonia that are equally high on hedonic enjoyment. The converse is not true; that is, a high percentage of activities high on hedonic enjoyment are not high on eudaimonia.

Intrinsic motivating activities can be predicted by at least three variables: (1) perceived importance of the activity (assessed by one-item reading: "Overall, how important is this activity to you in your life?" the endpoints of the scale are identified as "not at all important" and "extremely important"); (2) the perception that these activities advance personal potentials (assessed by two summed items embedded within a series of items with the stem: "To what extent does this activity provide you with each of the following types of opportunities?" The relevant completions are "the opportunity for me to develop my best potentials" and "the opportunity for me to make progress toward my goals"; each item is associated with a scale with the endpoints identified as "not at all" and "very extensively"), and (3) the amount of effort invested in these activities (assessed by one item reading: "What is the usual level of effort you invest when you engage in this activity?" The scale ranged from "very low" to "very high").

Like intrinsic motivation, personal expressiveness is linked to personal growth, a focal aspect of eudaimonia. The individual experiences personal growth mostly through engagement in activities that are personally expressive. The individual perceives that engagement in these activities are important life goals; these activities lead to realization of one's potential; and they require an investment of resources (time, effort, and perhaps money). As such, one can argue that eudaimonia may involve a preponderance of manifestations of intrinsic motivation (expressions related to personal expressiveness plus hedonia) relative to manifestations of extrinsic motivation (expressions related to hedonia alone). Personal expressiveness research supports the definition of positive balance at the developmental level. That is, well-being and positive mental health at the developmental level involve a preponderance of positive psychological traits related to intrinsic motivation (i.e., personal expressiveness) relative to negative psychological traits related to extrinsic motivation (i.e., hedonia alone).

Psychological Well-Being

Ryff's (1989) concept of psychological well-being captures the best conceptualization of eudaimonia. Psychological well-being is essentially personal growth and development. The construct of psychological well-being involves personal growth, purpose in life, environmental mastery, autonomy, and positive relations with others (cf. Ryff and Keyes 1995; Ryff & Singer, 1996, 1998, 2008). See measure in Table 6.2.

Table 6.2 Ryff's psychological well-being measure

Autonomy

  • I am not afraid to voice my opinions even when they are in opposition to the opinions of most people.

    • My decisions are not usually influenced by what everyone else is doing.

    • I have confidence in my opinions even if they are contrary to the general consensus.

    • Being happy with myself is more important than having others approve of me.

    • I tend to worry what other people think of me. (reverse coded)

    • I often change my mind about decisions if my friends and family disagree. (reverse coded)

    • It is difficult for me to voice my own opinions on controversial matters. (reverse coded)

Positive relations with others

    • Most people see me as loving and affectionate.

    • I enjoy personal and mutual conversations with family members or friends.

    • People would describe me as a giving person, willing to share my time with others.

    • I know that I can trust my friends and they know that they can trust me.

    • I often feel lonely because I have few close friends with whom to share my concerns. (reverse coded)

    • I don't have many people who want to listen when I need to talk. (reverse coded)

    • It seems to me that most other people have more friends than I do. (reverse coded)

Environmental mastery

    • I am quite good at managing the many responsibilities of my daily life.

    • I generally do a good job of taking care of my personal finances and affairs.

    • I am good at juggling my time so that I can fit everything in that needs to be done.

    • I have been able to build a home and a lifestyle for myself that is to my liking.

    • I do not fir very well with the people and the community around me. (reverse coded)

    • I often feel overwhelmed by my responsibilities. (reverse coded)

    • I have difficulty arranging my life in a way that is satisfying to me. (reverse coded)

Personal growth

    • I think it is important to have new experiences that challenge how you think about the world.

    • I have the sense that I have developed a lot as a person over time.

    • I am not interested in activities that expand my horizons. (reverse coded)

    • I don't want to try new ways of doing things—my life is fine the way it is. (reverse coded)

    • When I think about it, I haven't really improved much as a person over the years. (reverse coded)

    • I do not enjoy being in new situations that require me to change my old familiar ways to doing things. (reverse coded)

    • There is a truth in the saying that you can't teach an old dog new tricks. (reverse coded)

Purpose in life

    • I am an active person in carrying out the plans I set for myself.

    • I enjoy making plans for the future and working to make them a reality.

    • I tend to focus on the present, because the future nearly always brings me problems. (reverse coded)

    • My daily activities often seem trivial and unimportant to me. (reverse coded)

    • I don't have a good sense of what it is I am trying to accomplish in life. (reverse coded)

    • I used to set goals for myself, but that now seems a waste of time. (reverse coded)

Response scale: Responses are captured on 6-point Likert-type scales varying from 1 (strongly disagree) to 6 (strongly agree)

Source: Adapted from Abbott et al. (2010)

Ryff (2014) reviewed much of the research related to psychological well-being addressing neglected aspects of positive functioning such as purposeful engagement in life and realization of one's potential. In this seminal article, Ryff addressed a set of questions related to development across the life span, personality correlates, work and other community activities, health and biological risk factors, and clinical intervention.

How psychological well-being changes across adult development and later life? Research has shown that aging has been linked with higher psychological well-being overall but with notable declines in purpose in life and personal growth. Those who feel younger than they are, but do not wish to be younger, experience higher levels of psychological well-being. However, realism in self-evaluation (rather than illusion) predicts higher psychological well-being. Psychological well-being changes as people deal with the challenges of adult life, and improvements in psychological well-being seems to be associated with downward social comparisons, flexible self-perceptions, and the use of coping strategies.

What are the personality correlates of psychological well-being? Research has shown that psychological well-being is correlated with optimism, the use of life management strategies, intentional activities, empathy, and emotional intelligence.

How psychological well-being is linked with experiences in family life? Research has shown that greater role involvement promotes higher psychological well-being. Specifically, helping family members tend to enhance purpose and self-acceptance. Those who experience marriage longevity tend to report higher psychological well-being compared to the divorced, widowed or never married. However, single women who are high on autonomy tend to experience higher levels of personal growth compared to married women. Parenting tend to enhance psychological well-being among adults, particularly if one's children are doing well. Loss of a child in adulthood is associated with lower levels of psychological well-being decades later. Conversely, loss of a parent in childhood is associated with lower levels of psychological well-being in adulthood. Emotional and physical abuse in childhood compromises psychological well-being in adulthood. Interestingly, caring for an aging parent also is associated with declines in psychological well-being, although less so for daughters with high environmental mastery.

How psychological well-being relates to work and other community activities? The research indicates that psychological well-being contributes to, and is influenced by, various career pursuits. Psychological well-being also plays a role in work-life balance in that those high on well-being tend to experience less work-family conflict, especially among younger cohorts of both men and women. How work and family influence psychological well-being seem to be moderated by culture too. Volunteering, among the elderly, is associated with higher psychological well-being. Moreover, religiosity is associated with higher levels of purpose and growth but lower levels of autonomy.

What are the connections between psychological well-being and health? Research shows that psychological well-being is compromised among those with illnesses and disabilities. Interestingly, the research also shows that individuals high on purpose in life benefit from reduced risk of stroke and myocardial infarction.

Other research has linked aspects of psychological well-being to health behaviors such as exercise, sleep, and weight maintenance. Studies have also shown that higher levels of psychological well-being are associated with better biological regulation in terms of stress hormones, inflammatory markers, and cardiovascular risk factors. These benefits still hold despite risk associated with low socioeconomic status. Studies from neuroscience provide evidence showing that those with higher psychological well-being experience less amygdala activation and more engagement of higher-order cortical structures when exposed to negative stimuli. When exposed to positive stimuli, individuals with higher psychological well-being experience sustained activation of the reward circuitry and reduced levels of stress hormones. In sum, psychological well-being seems to serve adaptive, protective functions in relation to health and disease.

How psychological well-being can be promoted for ever-greater segments of society via clinical and intervention programs? Ryff asserts that mental disorders (schizophrenia, depression, panic disorder, cyclothymia, agoraphobia, post-traumatic stress disorder, etc.) tend to compromise the individual's sense of mastery, growth, purpose and positive self-regard, important aspects of psychological well-being. Conversely, research shows that high levels of psychological well-being sometimes mitigate symptoms of mental disorders. Improvement in psychological well-being is now recognized as an effective clinical treatment targets designed to prevent relapse. That is, the research provides much evidence suggesting that psychotherapy can be more effective when accompanied by interventions that enhance psychological well-being. Other interventions in schools and the workplace have demonstrated that programs to enhance psychological well-being can prevent mental illness and promote resilience.

The point of this discussion is to argue that positive psychological traits as captured by the five dimensions of psychological well-being (personal growth, purpose in life, environmental mastery, autonomy, and positive relations with others) are associated with a higher level construct of well-being, a construct that build on life satisfaction to include aspects of growth and intrinsic motivation. As such, one can argue that eudaimonia may involve a preponderance of positive psychological traits (e.g., personal growth, purpose in life, environmental mastery, autonomy, and positive relations with others) relative to negative traits (e.g., pessimism, hopelessness, helplessness, neuroticism, impulsiveness). Research on psychological well-being supports the definition of positive balance at the developmental level. That is, well-being and positive mental health at the developmental level involve a preponderance of positive psychological traits related to Ryff's dimensions of psychological well-being relative to negative traits.

Purpose and Meaning in Life

Well-being researchers have shown that the concept of purpose and meaning in life plays a very important role in subjective well-being. They refer to ideas developed by Victor Frankl (1963, 1967) and the panoply of subsequent writings (e.g. Steger et al., 2006). Much of this work support the notion that purpose and meaning are beneficial to human functioning. People who are aware of what life aspects are most vital and manage their lives consistently with those values are likely to experience high levels of subjective well-being. This construct has three dimensions, namely coherence, purpose, and significance (Martela & Steger, 2016). Coherence refers to a sense of comprehension that one's life make sense. Purpose refers to a sense of core goals, aims, and direction in life. Significance refers to a sense of life's inherent value and having a life worth living.

Examples of well-being measures based on the concept of purpose and meaning in life include the Meaning in Life Questionnaire-Presence Subscale (MLQ-P; Steger et al., 2006). The MLQ-P measure captures the degree to which people feel their lives are meaningful through five items (e.g., "I have a good sense of what makes my life meaningful"). Responses to each item are captured on a 7-point rating scale varying from "1 = absolutely untrue" to "7 = absolutely true." More recently, Schulenberg and Melton (2010) have provided some evidence of construct validity to the Purpose-in-Life (PIL) measure (Chamberlain & Zika, 1988; Dyck, 1987; Hicks & King, 2007; Melton & Schulenberg, 2008; Morgan & Farsides, 2009). Respondents express the extent to which they feel enthusiasm in living, whether they feel life is exciting, if they have clear life goals, whether the life they live has been worthwhile, whether they have a reason for being alive, whether the world is meaningful, and whether they feel they have a life purpose (cf. Schulenberg et al., 2011).

Extensive research has documented links between personality traits and well-being (DeNeve & Cooper, 1998). In this context, there is empirical evidence that meaning in life contributes to psychological well-being (e.g., Ryff, 1989). Evidence also suggests that the construct is an important predictor of positive mental health (e.g., Halama & Dedova, 2007). Furthermore, several studies have shown that meaning in life is positively linked to life satisfaction (e.g., Zika & Chamberlain, 1992), self-esteem (e.g., Rathi & Rastogi, 2007), achievement motivation (e.g., Steger et al., 2008); and negatively related to depression and anxiety (e.g., Riichiro & Masahiko, 2006).

The preceding discussion indicates that purpose and meaning in life is a positive psychological trait and an important element of eudaimonic well-being. As such, one can argue that eudaimonia may involve a preponderance of positive psychological traits (e.g., purpose and meaning in life) relative to negative traits (e.g., pessimism, hopelessness, helplessness, neuroticism, impulsiveness). Research on purpose and meaning in life supports the definition of positive balance at the developmental level. That is, well-being and positive mental health at the developmental level involve a preponderance of positive psychological traits that include purpose and meaning in life relative to negative traits.

Authentic Happiness and Orientations to Happiness

To reiterate, Haybron (2000) made the distinction among three philosophical concepts of happiness: psychological happiness, prudential happiness, and perfectionist happiness. These three philosophical approaches to happiness (psychological, prudential, and perfectionist) are highly akin to Seligman's (2002) distinction of the pleasant life (psychological happiness), the engaged life (prudential happiness), and the meaningful life (perfectionist happiness). This is Seligman's view of the concept he calls "authentic happiness." In other words, authentic happiness comes about as a function of meeting three major needs: the need to have a pleasant life (pleasure), the need to have an engaged life (engagement), and the need to have a meaningful life (virtue). The pleasant life is about happiness in a hedonic sense. The engaged life is about happiness through engagement. The meaningful life is about happiness by achieving virtue.

The *need to have a pleasant life* is based on Seligman's interpretation of *hedonism*, which is a matter of maximizing feelings of pleasure and minimizing feelings of pain. Hedonism has its modern conceptual roots in Bentham's utilitarianism and its manifestation in American consumerism. Seligman points to the research by Danny Kahneman (the Nobel Prize winner in behavioral economics) as an example of happiness conceptualized in terms of the Pleasant Life. According to Kahneman (1999), happiness is essentially momentary experiences of pleasures. Kahneman uses the *Experience Sampling Method* (ESM) to measure happiness. This method involves having researchers beep their subjects at random during the day asking how much pleasure or pain they are experiencing at the moment. Based on these momentary perceptions of positive and negative affect, Kahneman computes approximate total happiness points over the week. Thus, happiness as "objective happiness" for a given time period is computed by adding up subjects' on-line hedonic assessments of all the individual moments that comprise that period. Seligman's *theory of authentic happiness* considers hedonism in that part of what makes a happy life pleasant. Happiness in the present involves paying attention to bodily pleasures and enhancing these pleasures. The author provides good advice on how people can enhance their pleasures through habituation (i.e., spreading out the events that produce pleasure far enough to generate a craving), savoring (i.e., indulging the senses), and mindfulness (i.e., becoming acutely aware of the surrounding).

In contrast, the *need to have an engaged life* refers to gratification, not pleasure. Engagement in life goes beyond hedonism. Happiness in the context of the engaged life is a matter of getting what you want. The engaged life holds that fulfillment of a *desire* contributes to one's happiness regardless of the amount of pleasure (or displeasure). Desire may be in the form of wanting truth, illumination, and purity. These desires are very different from bodily pleasures. Happiness through engagement in life moves from hedonism's amount of pleasure felt to the somewhat less subjective state of how well one is engaged/absorbed and how well one's desires are satisfied. Seligman provides plenty of advice to his readers on how to enhance

Table 6.3 Orientations to happiness

The pleasant life
− Life is too short to postpone the pleasures it can provide.
− I go out of my way to feel euphoric.
− In choosing what I do, I always take into account whether it will be pleasurable.
− I agree with the statement: "Life is short—eat dessert first."
− I love to do things that excite my senses.
− For me, the good life is the pleasurable life.

The engaged life
− Regardless of what I am doing, time passes very quickly.
− I seek out situations that challenge my skills and abilities.
− Whether at work or play, I am usually "in a zone" and not conscious of myself.
− I am always very absorbed in what I do.
− In choosing what to do, I always take into account whether I can lose myself in it.
− I am rarely distracted by what is going on around me.

The meaningful life
− My life serves a higher purpose.
− In choosing what to do, I always take into account whether it will benefit other people.
− I have a responsibility to make the world a better place.
− My life has a lasting meaning.
− What I do matters to society.
− I have spent a lot of time thinking about what life means and how I fit in the big picture.

Response scale: 5-point rating scale varying from 1 = "very much unlike me" to 5 = "very much like me"
Source: Adapted from Chen (2010, p. 435)

gratification by engaging in activities that generate flow experience. Thus, in addition to experiencing pleasure (the pleasant life), people can experience desire fulfillment through engagement (the engaged life).

Finally, with respect to the *need to have a meaningful life*, Seligman maintains that happiness consists of a human life that achieves certain things from a list of worthwhile pursuits such as career accomplishments, friendship, freedom from disease and pain, material comforts, civic spirit, beauty, education, love, knowledge, and good conscience. Thus, leading a meaningful life is key to happiness. The meaningful life is not necessarily subjective as is the pleasant life (and the engaged life). Leading a meaningful life is objective. The person who lives a meaningful life is one that serves what is larger and more worthwhile than just the self's pleasures and desires.

Peterson et al. (2005) developed a measure based on Seligman's theory of authentic happiness (cf. Chen, 2010; Peterson et al., 2007; Vella-Brodrick et al. 2009). The measure is captured in Table 6.3 and seems to capture the three major dimensions of happiness—hedonic well-being, life satisfaction, and eudaimonia. Of course, our interest in this chapter is eudaimonia; that is, the third dimension of orientation to happiness. The same authors conducted two studies to test the notion that people who score highly on the three dimensions of authentic happiness (life of pleasure, life of engagement, and life of meaning) score high on traditional measures of life satisfaction, and vice versa. The first study involved adult volunteers who participated in an on-line survey. The goal of the study was to develop the measures capturing the three dimensions of authentic happiness. The second study, also respondents who completed an on-line survey, shows that respondents scoring simultaneously high on all three dimensions reported significantly higher life satisfaction than those who scored low on the same dimensions. Thus, these results provide some support for Seligman's theory of authentic happiness.

The preceding discussion indicates that authentic happiness, *a la* Seligman, is a higher-order construct akin to eudaiomina. The key dimension of authentic happiness that corresponds directly to eudaimonia is the meaningful life; the other two dimensions (the pleasant life and the engaged life) are subsumed within this higher-order construct. As such, one can argue that eudaimonia may involve a preponderance of positive psychological traits (e.g., the meaningful life) relative to negative traits (e.g., pessimism, hopelessness, helplessness, neuroticism, impulsiveness). Research on authentic happiness supports the definition of positive balance at the developmental level. That is, well-being and positive mental health at the developmental level involve a preponderance of positive psychological traits that include the meaningful life relative to negative traits.

Flourishing

In 2011, Seligman wrote another book called *Flourish: A Visionary New Understanding of Happiness and Well-Being* (Seligman, 2011). In that book, he revised his theory of authentic happiness as follows. The focus of the authentic happiness theory is on happiness, operationalized using a variety of life satisfaction self-report measures. Seligman argues that life satisfaction measures are essentially reflective in the sense that the construct is customarily measured using multiple indicators. The new theory of flourishing captures well-being in totality, both objectively and subjectively. Well-being is not operationalized through reflective measures of life satisfaction. Well-being, in this case, is a latent construct captured by its determinants, namely PERMA (**P**ositive emotions, **E**ngagement, positive **R**elationships, **M**eaning, and **A**ccomplishment) through a formative measure. In other words, the concept of well-being comprises five elements, and the measurement of the elements reflects the totality of well-being of an individual.

Authentic happiness occurs as a function of three major determinants: pleasant life, engaged life, and meaningful life. In contrast, the theory of flourishing builds on the theory of authentic happiness by including the first three determinants (the pleasant life addressed in the new theory as **P**ositive emotions, the engaged life addressed in the new theory as **E**ngagement, and the meaningful life addressed in the new theory as **M**eaning).

The fourth element of well-being is positive **R**elationships. People pursue social connectedness, and this goal is essentially an end goal. People do not connect with others for the sake of attaining other goals. That is not to say that in some cases seeking and maintaining positive relationships with others do not help the individual attain other goals. Positive relationships can also serve as a means to an end.

Table 6.4 The flourishing scale

• I lead a purposeful and meaningful life.
• My social relationships are supportive and rewarding.
• I am engaged and interested in my daily activities.
• I actively contribute to the happiness and well-being of others.
• I am competent and capable in the activities that are important to me.
• I am a good person and live a good life.
• I am optimistic about my future.
• People treat me with respect

Response scale: Responses are recorded on a 7-point Likert-type scale varying from 1 (strongly disagree) to 7 (strongly agree)
Source: Adapted from Diener et al. (2010)

However, Seligman emphasized that we are inherently social animals, and as such we seek positive relationships as an end goal—a terminal value. Loneliness is profoundly a disabling condition among humans, and the pursuit of positive connections with others is a fundamental human need.

The last element of well-being (**A**ccomplishment) refers to the tendency that people pursue success, accomplishment, winning, mastery, and achievement for their own sakes. In other words, these are terminal values, not instrumental values. Accomplishment is pursued for its own sake even if it does not induce positive emotions upon goal attainment. It is the thrill of the game (or accomplishment), rather than the positive emotions associated with winning the game.

The concept of "flourishing" has been captured through the *Flourishing Scale* (Diener et al., 2010). This is a brief 8-item summary measure of the respondent's self-perceived success in important areas such as relationships, self-esteem, purpose, and optimism. Table 6.4 shows the measure.

The preceding discussion indicates that PERMA concept is a higher order construct akin to eudaimonia. The key dimensions of PERMA that correspond directly to eudaimonia is **M**eaning, positive **R**elationships, and **A**ccomplishment; the other two dimensions (**P**ositive emotions and **E**ngagement) are subsumed within this higher-order construct. As such, one can argue that eudaimonia may involve a preponderance of positive psychological traits (e.g., positive emotions, engagement, meaning, positive relationships, and accomplishment) relative to negative traits (e.g., pessimism, hopelessness, helplessness, neuroticism, impulsiveness). Research on the PERMA model supports the definition of positive balance at the developmental level. That is, well-being and positive mental health at the developmental level involve a preponderance of positive psychological traits relative to negative traits.

Resilience

Some people are more resilient than others. When they first experience adversity, their well-being suffers on temporarily; after which they bounce back. That is, their well-being bounces back to its set point. In other words, they recover the normal pattern after they have been disrupted. Thus, resilience is viewed as an ability to recover from or adjust easily to misfortune or change. Cummins and Wooden (2014) argue that resilience reflects the power of homeostasis to retain an adaptive level of well-being and to restore the normal level of well-being following a negative deviation caused by an adverse circumstance.

Much evidence suggests that some children raised in adverse circumstances are more resilient than others (e.g., Masten & Coatsworth, 1998, Werner & Smith, 1982). The research also points out that the process of recovery and adjustment requires resources, both mental and physical resources. Resources may include supportive relationships, external to the individual as well as resources internal to the person, such as being meaningfully connected to at least one other person, and that one's life is under control (e.g., Werner, 1995). These eudaimonic traits, not only do they provide positive resources in their own right, but also raise the probability that future stress can be mitigated. As such eudaimonia is treated as a mental resource (Masten, 2007); the greater the eudaimonic well-being the greater the resilience.

Satisfaction of the Full Spectrum of Human Needs

Seligman's (2011) PERMA model has a certain affinity to Maslow's (1954/1970) hierarchy of needs. One can argue that Positive emotions, or hedonic well-being, is a concept reflective of satisfaction of physiological needs. Eating, drinking, and having sex produce visceral-level happiness. Engagement can be viewed through the lens of the need for esteem. People engage in various activities to gain status within their immediate and extended communities. Positive Relationships can be viewed in terms of social needs. People are motivated to gain approval and avoid disapproval from significant others. Meaning may reflect aspects of growth-related needs such as self-actualization, knowledge, and aesthetics. Similarly, Accomplishment could be viewed as overlapping with the need to self-actualize, which manifests itself in terms of environmental mastery.

As such, one can argue that true happiness is experienced when the individual experiences satisfaction with basic needs (e.g., biological needs, safety needs, and economic needs), as well as growth needs (e.g., social, esteem, self-actualization, knowledge, and aesthetic needs) (cf. Sirgy & Wu, 2009).

My colleagues and I (Sirgy et al., 1995) developed a measure of happiness based on Maslow's need hierarchy theory. Four need categories were used (survival needs, social needs, ego needs, and self-actualization needs). The items are shown in Table 6.5.

At a more macro level, my colleagues and I used the same theoretical perspective to conceptualize quality of life and national development (Sirgy, 1986; Sirgy & Mangleburg, 1988). We argued that quality of life can be better met at the national level by considering the level of economic development of a country and the needs of most of the people in that country. Therefore, in economically developed

Table 6.5 A need satisfaction hierarchy measure of well-being

- The feeling of having been secure
- The feeling of having given to (and having received help from) others
- The feeling of having developed close friendships
- The feeling of having been 'in the know'
- The feeling of self-esteem (pride) a person has about oneself
- The feeling of prestige (reputation) one person has about oneself
- The feeling of having experienced independent thought and action
- The feeling of having determined my life course
- The feeling of having experienced personal growth and development
- The feeling of having experienced self-fulfillment
- The feeling of having had worthwhile accomplishments

The following scales are used to record responses for each of the 11 items:
How much is there now?
Minimum 1 2 3 4 5 6 7 Maximum
How much should there be?
Minimum 1 2 3 4 5 6 7 Maximum

The overall score of life satisfaction of a respondent is computed by taking the absolute difference score (between "how much is there now" and "how much should there be") for each item and deriving an average score. The lower the resultant average score, the higher the overall life satisfaction.

Source: Adapted from Sirgy et al. (1995)

countries, policies should be created to encourage the implementation of economic policies designed to meet higher-order needs. Conversely, for the less-developed countries, policies should target lower-order needs mostly.

More recently the same theme was echoed by Tov and Diener (2009). They asserted that countries that do not meet the basic needs of their citizens suffer from ill-being. They rate low on measures of subjective well-being (cf. Diener, Diener, & Diener, 1995). Once basic needs are generally met, higher-order needs (e.g., self-development and social relationships) gain prominence. This may explain why income is more strongly correlated in developing than developed countries (Diener & Diener, 1995; Oishi et al., 1999).

The preceding discussion indicates that eudaimonia can be construed through a composite of motivational constructs inherent in Maslow's hierarchy of needs. High levels of eudaimonic well-being occur as a direct function of satisfaction of the full spectrum of basic and growth needs, *a la* Maslow. The need satisfaction construct is a higher-order construct that not only captures growth-related traits but also traits related to basic needs. As such, one can argue that eudaimonia may involve a preponderance of positive psychological traits (e.g., satisfaction of both basic and growth needs) relative to negative traits (e.g., pessimism, hopelessness, helplessness, neuroticism, impulsiveness). Research on the need satisfaction model supports the definition of positive balance at the developmental level. That is, well-being and positive mental health at the developmental level involve a preponderance of positive psychological traits relative to negative traits.

Emergence

Eudaimonia is a well-being concept best understood in the context of the hierarchy of concepts of well-being at the developmental level—the focal point of this chapter. As such, the reader is now in a better position to appreciate the link between well-being at the meta-cognitive level and that at the developmental level. How does well-being at the meta-cognitive level (i.e., life satisfaction) contribute to the formation of well-being at the developmental level (i.e., eudaimonia)? As presented in the preceding chapters, this link can be viewed in terms of emergence—a concept well-entrenched in systems science. To further reiterate, emergence refers to higher-level systems "emerge" from lower-level systems. Complex systems have "emergent properties" that are not inherent in their individual parts and cannot be understood even with full understanding of the parts alone. Much research demonstrates a strong relationship between global judgments of life satisfaction and various measures of eudaimonic well-being. Here is suggestive evidence. Research has shown that there is a positive association between the life satisfaction judgments and measures of psychological well-being (e.g., Compton et al., 1996; Joshanloo et al., 2018a, b; Kafka & Kozma, 2002; Kardas et al., 2019; Keyes et al., 2002; Ryff and Keyes, 1995; Sanjuan, 2011; Waterman, 2007; Wilson & Somhlaba, 2016). Factor analyses also show that psychological well-being and life satisfaction measures are distinct from each other (e.g., Compton, 1998; Compton et al., 1996; Kafka & Kozma, 2002; Keyes et al., 2002).

Evidence is also available relating positive life evaluations with specific dimensions of eudaimonia. Examples include:

- *Self-acceptance*, a well-established dimension of eudaimonia, is positive related with life satisfaction (Abd-Al-Atty et al., 2010).
- There is also evidence suggesting a significant relationship between life satisfaction judgments and measures of *personal growth*, a well-established dimension of eudaimonia (Stevic & Ward, 2008).
- There is also evidence suggesting a significant relationship between life satisfaction judgments and measures of *purpose in life*, another dimension of eudaimonia (e.g., Ang & Jiaging, 2012).
- Evidence exists linking life satisfaction judgments with *personal autonomy*, another dimension of eudaimonia (e.g., Chai, Kowk, & Gu, 2018).
- Additionally, there is evidence linking life satisfaction judgments with measures of *positive relations with others*, yet another dimension of eudaimonia (e.g., Segrin & Rynes, 2009).

The antonyms of eudaimonia include pessimism, hopelessness, depressive disorders, and neuroticism. As such, there is also evidence suggesting that these negative personality traits characteristics are negatively related to judgments of life satisfaction: pessimism (e.g., Luger, Cotter, & Sherman, 2009), hopelessness (e.g., Karatas, Aslan, & Bascillar, 2019), depressive disorders (e.g., Lee, Choi, & Lee, 2019), and neuroticism (e.g., Liang, 2015).

The preceding discussion points to the possibility that life satisfaction at the meta-cognitive level interacts with other variables in a psychological process related to personal growth and intrinsic motivation to produce a new well-being phenomenon at the developmental level, namely eudaimonia. That is, life satisfaction seems to be a *necessary but not sufficient* ingredient of eudaimonia. It is a building block in the formation of eudaimonia. For a person to experience high levels of eudaimonic well-being, he or she must also experience high levels of life satisfaction. The person then must be involved with experiences related to person growth and intrinsic motivation. The resultant outcome is eudaimonia as reflected in a set of personal strength such as character strength, self-acceptance, purpose in life, environmental mastery, autonomy, positive relations with others, among others. In sum, *life satisfaction at the meta-cognitive level mediated by a process involving high personal growth result in high levels of eudaimonia at the developmental level; and conversely, life dissatisfaction mediated by a process involving low personal growth result into low levels of eudaimonia* (see Fig. 6.1).

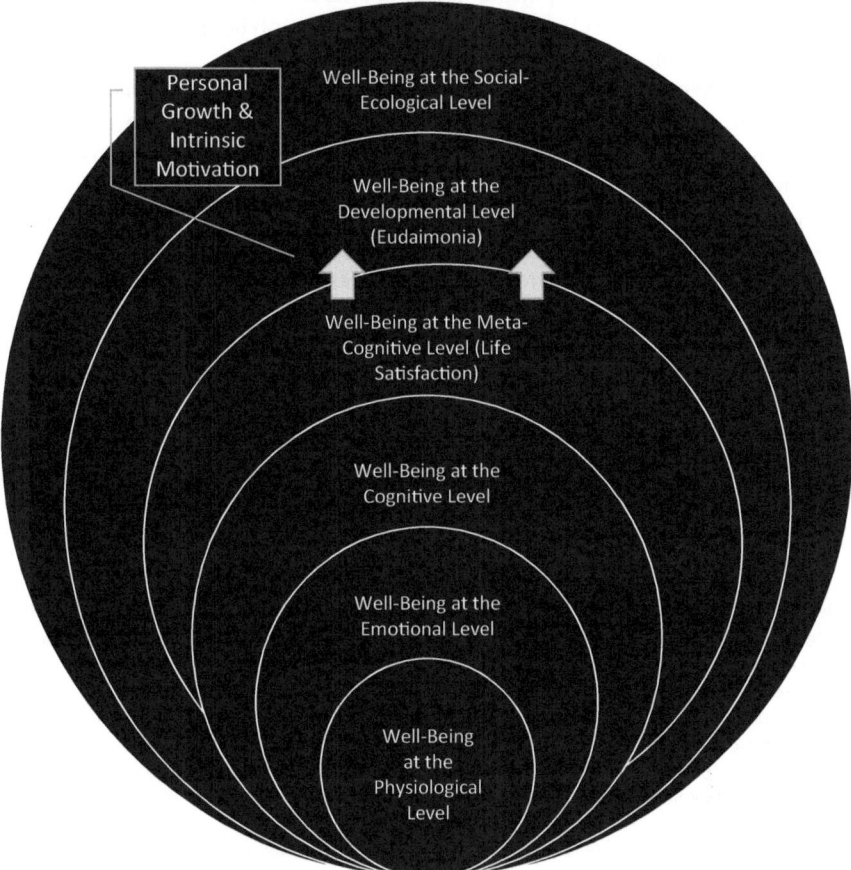

Fig. 6.1 Emergence: Well-being at the developmental level (Eudaimonia) influenced by well-being at the meta-cognitive level (life satisfaction) mediated by a process of personal growth and intrinsic motivation

Conclusion

I presented a definition of positive mental health based on the concept of positive balance at the developmental level in this chapter. This definition is stated as follows: Individuals experiencing a preponderance of positive psychological traits (personal growth, purpose in life, environmental mastery, autonomy, positive relations with others, etc.) relative to negative psychological traits (pessimism, hopelessness, depressive disorder, neuroticism, impulsiveness, etc.). I then discussed nine programs of research, supporting this definition: hedonic versus eudaimonic happiness; virtue ethics and balance; self-determination theory; personal expressiveness; psychological well-being; purpose and meaning in life; authentic happiness and orientations to happiness; flourishing; resilience, and satisfaction of the full spectrum of human needs. Following this discussion, I described how positive balance expressed in eudaimonia (at the developmental level) is produced in part by life satisfaction (at the meta-cognitive level) mediated by a process involving personal growth and intrinsic motivation.

The next chapter focuses on positive balance as viewed from the most superordinate level of analysis, namely the social-ecological level. I have coined this phenomenon, "socio-eudaimonia" to capture well-being that has elements of both eudaimonia (at the developmental level) and social functioning (at the social-ecological level). A definition of positive balance at the social-ecological level is then discussed. This definition is stated as follows: Individuals experiencing a preponderance of social resources (social acceptance, social actualization, social contribution, social integration, etc.) relative to social constraints (social exclusion, ostracism, etc.). I then discuss six programs of research supporting this definition: social well-being, need to belong, attachment theory, social ostracism, and social harmony.

References

Abbott, R. A., Ploubidis, G. B., Huppert, F. A., Kuh, D., & Croudace, T. J. (2010). An evaluation of the precision of measurement of Ryff's psychological well-being scales in a population sample. *Social Indicators Research, 97*, 357–373.

Abd-Al-Atty, M. F., Mohamed, H.-A. E., Abdellah, A. F., Farid, T. M., & Mortagy, A. K. (2010). Self-acceptance and life satisfaction in Egyptian older people: Can one exist without the other? *Australasian Journal on Ageing, 29*, 183–184.

Ang, R. P., & Jiaqing, O. (2012). Association between caregiving, meaning in life, and life satisfaction beyond 50 in an Asian sample: Age as a moderator. *Social Indicators Research, 108*, 525–543.

Chai, W. Y., Kwok, S. Y. C. L., & Gu, M. (2018). Autonomy-granting parenting and child depression: The moderating roles of hope and life satisfaction. *Journal of Child and Family Studies, 27*, 2596–2607.

Chamberlain, K., & Zika, S. (1988). Measuring meaning in life: An examination of three scales. *Personality and Individual Differences, 9*, 589–596.

Chen, G.-H. (2010). Validating the orientations to Happiness Scale in a Chinese Sample of University Students. *Social Indicators Research, 99*, 431–442.

Compton, W. (1998). Measures of mental health and a five-factor theory of personality. *Psychological Reports, 83*, 371–381.

Compton, W., Smith, M., Cornish, K., & Qualls, D. (1996). Factor structure of mental health measures. *Journal of Personality and Social Psychology, 71*, 406–413.

Cummins, R. A., & Wooden, M. (2014). Personal resilience in times of crisis: The implications of SWB homeostasis and setpoints. *Journal of Happiness Studies, 15*, 223–235.

Deci, E. L., & Ryan, R. M. (1985). *Intrinsic motivation and self-determination in human behavior.* New York: Plenum.

Deci, E. L., & Ryan, R. M. (2008). Hedonia, eudaimonia, and well-being: An introduction. *Journal of Happiness Studies, 9*, 1–11.

Delle Fave, A., Brdar, I., Freire, T., Vella-Brodrick, D., & Wissing, M. P. (2011). The eudaimonic and hedonic components of happiness: Qualitative and quantitative findings. *Social Indicators Research, 100*, 185–207.

Demir, M., Ozen, A., Dogan, A., Bilyk, N. A., & Tyrell, F. A. (2011). I matter to my friend, therefore I am happy: Friendship, mattering, and happiness. *Journal of Happiness Studies, 12*, 983–1005.

DeNeve, K. M., & Cooper, H. (1998). The happy personality: A meta-analysis of 137 personality traits and subjective well-being. *Psychological Bulletin, 124*, 197–229.

Diener, E. (1984). Subjective well-being. *Psychological Bulletin, 95*, 542–575.

Diener, E., & Diener, M. (1995). Cross-cultural correlates of life satisfaction and self-esteem. *Journal of Personality and Social Psychology, 68*, 653–663.

Diener, E., Diener, M., & Diener, C. (1995). Factors predicting the subjective well-being of nations. *Journal of Personality and Social Psychology, 69*, 851–864.

Diener, E., Suh, E. M., Lucas, R. E., & Smith, H. L. (1999). Subjective well-being: Three decades of progress. *Psychological Bulletin, 125*, 276–302.

Diener, E., Wirtz, D., Tov, W., Kim-Prieto, C., Choi, D., Oishi, S., et al. (2010). New well-being measures: Short scales to assess flourishing and positive and negative feelings. *Social Indicators Research, 97*, 143–156.

Duckworth, A. L., & Gross, J. J. (2014). Self-control and grit: Related but separable determinants of success. *Current Directions in Psychological Science, 23*, 319–325.

Dyck, M. J. (1987). Assessing logotherapeutic constructs: Conceptual and psychometric status of the purpose in life and seeking of noetic goals tests. *Clinical Psychology Review, 7*, 439–447.

Flückiger, C., & Grosse Holtforth, M. (2008). Focusing the therapist's attention on the patient's strengths: A preliminary study to foster a mechanism of change in outpatient psychotherapy. *Journal of Clinical Psychology, 64*, 876–890.

Frankl, V. (1963). *Man's search for meaning* (Revised ed.). London: Hodder & Stoughton.

Frankl, V. (1967). *Psychotherapy and existentialism.* New York: Simon & Schuster.

Halama, P., & Dedova, M. (2007). Meaning in life and hope as predictors of positive mental health: Do they explain residual variance not predicted by personality traits? *Studia Psychologica, 49*, 191–200.

Haybron, D. M. (2000). Two philosophical problems in the study of happiness. *Journal of Happiness Studies, 1*, 207–225.

Hicks, J. A., & King, L. A. (2007). Meaning in life and seeing the big picture: Positive affect and global focus. *Cognition and Emotion, 21*, 1577–1584.

Howell, R. T., Chenot, D., Hill, G., & Howell, C. J. (2011). Momentary happiness: The role of psychological need satisfaction. *Journal of Happiness Studies, 12*, 1–15.

Huppert, F. A. (2009). Psychological well-being: Evidence regarding its causes and consequences. *Applied Psychology: Health and Well-Being, 1*, 137–164.

Joshanloo, M. (2016). Revisiting the empirical distinction between hedonic and eudaimonic aspects of well-being using exploratory structural equation modeling. *Journal of Happiness Studies, 17*, 2023–2036.

Joshanloo, M., Sirgy, M. J., & Park, J. (2018a). Directionality of the relationship between social well-being and subjective well-being: Evidence from a 20-year longitudinal study. *Quality of Life Research, 27*, 2137–2145.

Joshanloo, M., Sirgy, M. J., & Park, J. (2018b). The importance of national levels of eudaimonic well-being to life satisfaction in old age: A global study. *Quality of Life Research, 27*, 3303–3311.

Kafka, G., & Kozma, A. (2002). The construct validity of Ryff's scales of psychological well-being (SPWB) and their relationship to measures of subjective well-being. *Social Indicator Research, 57*, 171–190.

Kahneman, D. (1999). Objective happiness. In D. Kahneman, E. Diener, & N. Schwartz (Eds.), *Well-Being: The foundations of hedonic psychology* (pp. 3–25). New York: Russell Sage Foundation.

Karatas, K., Aslan, H., & Bascillar, M. (2019). Hopelessness and satisfaction with wife among disabled veterans. *Journal of Society & Social Work, 30*, 1–18.

Kardas, F., Cam, Z., Eskisu, M., & Gelibou, S. (2019). Gratitude, hope, optimism and life satisfaction as predictors of psychological well-being. *Eurasian Journal of Educational Research (EJER), 82*, 81–100.

Kasser, T. (2016). Materialistic values and goals. *Annual Review of Psychology, 67*, 489–514.

Kesebir, P., & Diener, E. (2009). In pursuit of happiness: Empirical answers to philosophical questions. In E. Diener (Ed.), *The science of well-being: The collected works of Ed Diener* (pp. 59–74). Dordrecht, The Netherlands: Springer.

Keyes, C., Shmotkin, D., & Ryff, C. (2002). Optimizing well-being: The empirical encounter of two traditions. *Journal of Personality and Social Psychology, 82*, 1007–1022.

Lee, S.-W., Choi, J.-S., & Lee, M. (2019). Life satisfaction and depression in the oldest old: A longitudinal study. *International Journal of Aging & Human Development.* https://doi.org/10.1177/0091415019843448

Liang, H.-L. (2015). Testing a negative workplace event and life satisfaction in Taiwan: Neuroticisms as two moderators of the mediating roles of psychological strain. *Social Indicators Research, 120*, 559–583.

Luger, T., Cotter, K. A., & Sherman, A. M. (2009). It's all in how you view it: Pessimism, social relations, and life satisfaction in older adults with osteoarthritis. *Aging and Mental Health, 13*, 635–647.

Martela, F., & Steger, M. F. (2016). The three meanings of meaning in life: Distinguishing coherence, purpose, and significance. *The Journal of Positive Psychology, 11*, 531–545.

Maslow, A. H. (1954, 1970). *Motivation and personality.* New York: Harper.

Masten, A. S. (2007). Resilience in developing systems: Progress and promise as the fourth wave rises. *Development and Psychopathology, 19*, 921–930.

Masten, A. S., & Coatsworth, J. D. (1998). The development of competence in favorable and unfavorable environments: Lessons from research on successful children. *American Psychologist, 53*, 205–220.

Melton, A. M. A., & Schulenberg, S. E. (2008). On the measurement of meaning: Logotherapy's empirical contributions to Humanistic psychology. *The Humanistic Psychologist, 36*, 31–44.

Morgan, J., & Farsides, T. (2009). Measuring meaning in life. *Journal of Happiness Studies, 10*, 197–214.

Munoz Sastre, M. T. (1998). Lay conceptions of well-being and rules used in well-being judgements among young, middle-aged, and elderly adults. *Social Indicators Research, 47*, 203–231.

Niemiec, R. M. (2013). VIA character strengths: Research and practice (The first 10 years). In H. H. Knoop & A. Delle Fave (Eds.), *Well-being and cultures: Perspectives on positive psychology* (pp. 11–30). New York: Springer.

Oishi, S., Diener, E., Suh, E., & Lucas, R. E. (1999). The value as a moderator model in subjective well-being. *Journal of Personality, 67*, 157–183.

Park, N., & Peterson, C. (2009). Character strengths: Research and practice. *Journal of College and Character, 10*, 4.

Peterson, C., Park, N., & Seligman, M. E. P. (2005). Orientations to happiness and life satisfaction: The full life versus the empty life. *Journal of Happiness Studies, 6*, 24–41.

Peterson, C., Ruch, W., Beermann, U., Park, N., & Seligman, M. E. (2007). Strengths of character, orientations to happiness, and life satisfaction. *The Journal of Positive Psychology, 2*(3), 149–156.

Peterson, C., & Seligman, M. E. P. (2004). *Character strengths and virtues: A handbook of classification*. New York: Oxford University Press.

Quinlan, D., Swain, N., & Vella-Brodick, D. (2012). Character strengths interventions: Building on what we know for improved outcomes. *Journal of Happiness Studies, 13*, 1145–1163.

Rathi, N., & Rastogi, R. (2007). Meaning in life and psychological well-being in preadolescents and adolescents. *Journal of the Indian Academy of Applied Psychology, 33*, 31–38.

Riichiro, I., & Masahiko, O. (2006). Effects of a firm purpose in life on anxiety and sympathetic nervous activity caused by emotional stress: Assessment by psycho-physiological method. *Stress and Health, 22*, 275–281.

Rowe, C. J., & Broadie, S. (Eds.). (2002). *Nicomachean ethics*. Oxford: Oxford University Press.

Ryan, R. M., & Deci, E. L. (2000). Self-determination theory and the facilitation of instrinsic motivation, social development and well-being. *American Psychologist, 55*, 68–78.

Ryan, R. M., Huta, V., & Deci, E. L. (2008). Living well: A self-determination theory perspective on eudaimonia. *Journal of Happiness Studies, 9*, 139–170.

Ryff, C. D. (1989). Happiness is everything, or is it? Explorations on the meaning of psychological well-being. *Journal of Personality and Social Psychology, 57*, 1069–1081.

Ryff, C. (2014). Psychological well-being revisited: Advances in the science and practice of eudaimonia. *Psychotherapy and Psychosomatics, 83*, 10–28.

Ryff, C. D., & Keyes, C. L. M. (1995). The structure of psychological well-being revisited. *Journal of Personality and Social Psychology, 69*, 719–727.

Ryff, C. D., & Singer, B. (1996). Psychological well-being: Meaning, measurement, and implications for psychotherapy research. *Psychotherapy and Psychosomatics, 65*, 14–23.

Ryff, C. D., & Singer, B. (1998). The contours of positive human health. *Psychological Inquiry, 9*, 1–28.

Ryff, C. D., & Singer, B. (2008). Know thyself and become what you are: A Eudaimonic approach to psychological well-being. *Journal of Happiness Studies, 9*, 13–39.

Sanjuan, P. (2011). Affect balance as mediating variable between effective psychological functioning and satisfaction with life. *Journal of Happiness Studies, 12*, 373–384.

Schulenberg, S. E., & Melton, A. M. A. (2010). A confirmatory factor-analytic evaluation of the purpose in Life Test: Preliminary psychometric support for a replicable two-factor model. *Journal of Happiness Studies, 11*, 95–111.

Schulenberg, S. E., Schnetzer, L. W., & Buchanan, E. M. (2011). The purpose in life test-short form: Development and psychometric support. *Journal of Happiness Studies, 12*, 861–876.

Schwartz, B. (2015). *Why we work*. New York: Simon & Schuster.

Schwartz, B., & Wrzesniewski, A. (2016). Internal motivation, instrumental motivation, and Eudaimonia. In J. Vitterso (Ed.), *Handbook of eudaimonic well-being* (pp. 123–134). Dordrecht: Springer.

Segrin, C., & Rynes, K. N. (2009). The mediating role of positive relations with others in associations between depressive symptoms, social skills, and perceived stress. *Journal of Research in Personality, 43*, 962–971.

Seligman, M. E. P. (2002). *Authentic happiness: Using the new positive psychology to realize your potential for lasting fulfillment*. New York: The Free Press.

Seligman, M. E. P. (2011). *Flourish: A visionary new understanding of happiness and well-being*. New York: The Free Press.

Seligman, M. E. P. (2015). Chris Peterson's unfinished masterwork: The real mental illnesses. *The Journal of Positive Psychology, 10*, 3–6.

Seligman, M. E. P., Rashid, T., & Parks, A. C. (2006). Positive psychotherapy. *American Psychologist, 61*, 774–788.

Sirgy, M. J. (1986). A quality of life theory derived from Maslow's developmental perspective: "Quality" is related to progressive satisfaction of a hierarchy of needs, lower order and higher. *American Journal of Economics and Sociology, 45*(July), 329–342.

Sirgy, M. J., Cole, D., Kosenko, R., Meadow, H. L., Rahtz, D., Cicic, M., et al. (1995). Developing a life satisfaction measure based on need hierarchy theory. In M. J. Sirgy & A. C. Samli (Eds.), *New dimensions of marketing and quality of life* (pp. 3–26). Westport, CT: Greenwood Press.

Sirgy, M. J., & Mangleburg, T. M. (1988). Toward a general theory of social system development: A management/marketing perspective. *Systems Research, 5*, 115–130.

Sirgy, M. J., & Wu, J. (2009). The pleasant life, the engaged life, and the meaningful life: What about the balanced life? *Journal of Happiness Studies, 10*, 183–196.

Steger, M. F., Frazier, P., Oishi, S., & Kaler, M. (2006). The meaning in life questionnaire: Assessing the presence and search for meaning in life. *Journal of Counseling Psychology, 53*, 80–93.

Steger, M. F., Kashdan, T. B., Sullivan, B. A., & Lorentz, D. (2008). Understanding the search for meaning in life: Personality, cognitive style, and the dynamic between seeking and experiencing meaning. *Journal of Personality, 76*, 199–228.

Stevic, C. R., & Ward, R. M. (2008). Initiating personal growth: The role of recognition and life satisfaction on the development of college students. *Social Indicators Research, 89*, 523–547.

Tov, W., & Diener, E. (2009). The well-being of nations: Linking together trust, cooperation, and democracy. In E. Diener (Ed.), *The science of well-being: The collected works of Ed Diener* (pp. 155–173). Dordrecht, The Netherlands: Springer.

Vella-Brodrick, D. A., Park, N., & Peterson, C. (2009). Three ways to be happy: Pleasure, engagement, and meaning—findings from Australian and US samples. *Social Indicators Research, 90*, 165–179.

Vitterso, J. (Ed.). (2016). *Handbook of eudaimonic well-being.* Dordrecht: Springer.

Vitterso, J., Soholt, Y., Hetland, A., Alekseeva Thoresen, I., & Roysamb, E. (2010). Was Hercules happy? Some answers from a functional model of human well-being. *Social Indicators Research, 95*, 1–18.

Waterman, A. S. (1990). Personal expressiveness: Philosophical and psychological foundations. *Journal of Mind and Behaviour, 11*, 47–74.

Waterman, A. S. (1992). Identity as an aspect of optimal psychological functioning. In T. G. Adams & R. Montemayor (Eds.), *Advances in adolescent development* (Vol. 4, pp. 678–691). G. R. Newbury Park, CA: Sage.

Waterman, A. S. (1993). Two conceptions of happiness: Contrasts of personal expressiveness (eudaimonia) and hedonic enjoyment. *Journal of Personality and Social Psychology, 64*, 678–691.

Waterman, A. S. (2004). Finding someone to be: Studies on the role of intrinsic motivation in identity formation. *Identity: An International Journal of Theory and Research, 4*, 209–228.

Waterman, A. S. (2005). When effort is enjoyed: Two studies of intrinsic motivation for personally salient activities. *Motivation and Emotion, 29*, 165–188.

Waterman, A. S. (2007). Doing well: The relationships of identity status to three conceptions of well-being. *Identity: An International Journal of Theory and Research, 7*, 289–307.

Waterman, A. S., Schwartz, S. J., & Conti, R. (2008). The implications of two conceptions of happiness (hedonic enjoyment and eudaimonia) for the understanding of intrinsic motivation. *Journal of Happiness Studies, 9*, 41–79.

Waterman, A. S., Schwartz, S. J., Goldbacher, E., Green, H., Miller, C., & Philip, S. (2003). Predicting the subjective experience of intrinsic motivation: The roles of self-determination, the balance of challenges and skills, and self-realization values. *Personality and Social Psychology Bulletin, 29*, 1447–1458.

Werner, E. E. (1995). Resilience in development. *Current Directions in Psychological Science, 4*, 81–85.

Werner, E. E., & Smith, R. S. (1982). *Vulnerable but invincible: A longitudinal study of resilient children and youth.* New York: McGraw-Hill.

Wilson, A., & Somhlaba, N. Z. (2016). Psychological well-being in a context of adversity: Ghanaian adolescents' experiences of hope and life Satisfaction. *Africa Today, 63*(1), 84. Retrieved from http://search.ebscohost.com/login.aspx?direct=true&db=edspmu& AN=edspmu.S1527197816100105&site=eds-live&scope=site

Zika, S., & Chamberlain, K. (1992). On the relation between meaning in life and psychological well-being. *British Journal of Psychology, 83*, 133–145.

Chapter 7
Positive Balance at the Social-Ecological Level: Socio-Eudaimonia

Introduction

If our well-being depends upon the interaction between events in our brains and events in the world, and there are better and worse ways to secure it, then some cultures will tend to produce lives that are more worth living than others; some political persuasions will be more enlightened than others; and some world views will be mistaken in ways that cause needless human misery.—*Sam Harris, The Moral Landscape: How Science Can Determine Human Values* (https://www.goodreads.com/quotes/tag/well-being)

Robert E. Lane (1991, 1994, 1996, 2000), a political psychologist and a long-time quality-of-life scholar defines well-being as the relation between a person's subjective and objective sets of circumstances. The subjective set of circumstances reflecting high levels of subjective well-being involves nine elements:

1. capacity for enjoying life,
2. cognitive complexity,
3. a sense of autonomy and effectiveness,
4. self-knowledge,
5. self-esteem,
6. ease of interpersonal relations,
7. an ethical orientation,
8. personality integration, and
9. a productivity orientation.

Lane believes that these nine elements describing the psychological makeup of a person are the hallmark of mental health and social responsibility. These elements combined are responsible for a sense of overall well-being and social responsibility. This subjective set makes up what Lane calls the "quality of the person or QP."

© Springer Nature Switzerland AG 2020
M. J. Sirgy, *Positive Balance*, Social Indicators Research Series 80,
https://doi.org/10.1007/978-3-030-40289-1_7

The objective set reflects the quality of the environmental conditions (QC) representing opportunities for the person to use to achieve QP. Lane specifies nine opportunities and assets comprising a high quality of condition. These are:

1. Adequate material support;
2. Physical safety and security;
3. Available friends and social support;
4. Opportunities for the expression and receipt of love;
5. Opportunities for intrinsically challenging work;
6. Leisure opportunities that have elements of skill, creativity, and relaxation;
7. Available set of moral values that can give meaning to life;
8. Opportunities for self-development; and
9. Justice system that is managed by disinterested and competent parties.

Therefore, quality of life for an individual is essentially a direct function of the quality of the person and the quality of the conditions of the environment. In notation form,

$$QOL = f\,(QP, QC).$$

Why are Lane's ideas important? Lane makes the case that the concepts of well-being and positive mental health must consider both the psychology of well-being as reflected in the mind of the person *plus aspects of the environment* affecting the psychology of well-being. This is the essence of what I will be discussing in this chapter. I will describe the concept of socio-eudaimonia as the most superordinate construct of well-being by addressing aspects of eudaimonia in the context of the person's overall environment. People can be high on eudaimonia only if they well adapt to their environment. It is very likely that eudaimonic well-being would diminish given a non-supportive environment. Hence, eudaimonia plus a supportive environment help produce what is commonly referred to as "social well-being."

In the same vein, Carlquist, Ulleberg, Delle Fave, Nafstad, and Blakar (2017) made the case that perceptions of happiness and the good life can be categorized in terms of two key dimensions: internal and external. The external dimension involves a variety of happiness concepts related to social relationships, whereas the internal dimension focuses on the individual own emotional experiences. The effect of age was a key finding. Young people view happiness in relation to an internal conception of happiness, whereas older people view happiness in terms of the external dimension. In other words, as people age, their conception of happiness turns from inward to outward. This finding reinforces the notion that a holistic view of positive mental health should include both self and social dimensions. Bauer (2016) also emphasized the distinction between "internalist" and "externalist" beneficiaries of the good. The internalist beneficiary of the good mostly involves hedonic pleasures (i.e., positive and negative affect, life satisfaction, self-esteem, and hedonic motives) and eudaimonic meaning (i.e., psychological well-being, meaning in life, satisfaction of agentic needs, individual authenticity, and self-efficacy). In contrast, the externalist beneficiary of the good involves only eudaimonic meaning in the form of positive relations with others, social well-being, flourishing, satisfaction with communal needs, social authenticity, and identity status commitment.

As such, my definition of positive balance at the social-ecological level is: *Individuals experiencing a preponderance of social resources (social acceptance, social actualization, social contribution, social integration, social harmony, social belongingness, social attachment, familial attachment, etc.) relative to social constraints (social alienation, social discord, social exclusion, ostracism, etc.).* I will discuss several programs of research supporting this definition of well-being and how a process involving the development of social well-being plays an important role in establishing the ultimate state of well-being, "socio-eudaimonia." See the shaded are in Table 7.1 for a synopsis of this discussion.

Programs of Research Supporting the Positive Balance Definition

In the sections below I discuss five programs of research supporting the definition of positive mental health at the social-ecological level. These are: social well-being, social harmony, need to belong, attachment theory, and social exclusion and ostracism.

Social Well-being

Corey Keyes, a social psychologist from the sociology tradition, has made quite an impact in well-being research by advocating clearly a positive mental health perspective of mental well-being (Keyes, 1998). Specifically, he equates true happiness to positive mental health. Positive mental health involves feeling good and functioning well in society. He argues that positive mental health is flourishing in life, and the absence of positive mental health is languishing in life—key ingredients to eudaimonic well-being. Positive mental health is thus a syndrome of symptoms of both positive feelings and positive functioning in life and society. Keyes (2002) identified 13 dimensions of positive mental health:

1. Positive emotions,
2. Avowed satisfaction with life,
3. Environmental mastery (control),
4. Positive relations with others,
5. Personal growth,
6. Autonomy,
7. Having purpose in life,
8. Making a contribution to society,
9. Social integration,

Table 7.1 Positive mental health defined at various hierarchical levels as positive balance with emergence and focus on the social-ecological level

Level of analysis	Positive balance as positive mental health	Programs of research	Emergence
Positive mental health defined at a physiological level = **positive and negative neurotransmitters**	Individuals experiencing a preponderance of neurochemicals related to positive emotions (dopamine, serotonin, oxytocin) relative to neurochemicals related to negative emotions (cortisol)	Stress response system); neurobiology of happiness)	
Positive mental health defined at an emotional level = **positive/negative affect or hedonic well-being (positive/negative neurotransmitters + cognitive appraisals)**	Individuals experiencing a preponderance of positive emotions (happiness, joy, serenity, contentment, etc.) relative to negative emotions (anger, sadness, jealousy, envy, depression, etc.)	Positive versus negative affect; broaden and build theory; flow	Positive neurochemicals (dopamine, serotonin, and oxytocin) at the physiological level mediated by a process of cognitive appraisal (positive frame) result into positive affect (happiness, joy, contentment, etc.) at the emotional level; and conversely, negative neurochemicals (cortisol) mediated by a process of cognitive appraisal (negative frame) result into negative affect (anger, sadness, jealousy, envy, depression, etc.)
Positive mental health defined at a cognitive level = **domain satisfaction (positive/negative affect + domain segmentation)**	Individuals experiencing a preponderance of domain satisfaction (satisfaction in salient and multiple life domains such as family life, work life, social life, etc.) relative to dissatisfaction in other life domains	Principle of satisfaction limits; principle of the full spectrum of human developmental needs; principle of diminishing satisfaction	Positive affect (happiness, joy, contentment, etc.) at the emotional level mediated by a process of domain segmentation result into domain satisfaction (satisfied with work life, social life, family life, etc.); and conversely, negative affect (anger, sadness, jealousy, envy, depression, etc.) mediated by a process of domain segmentation result into domain dissatisfaction (dissatisfied with work life, social life, family life, etc.)
Positive mental health defined at a meta-cognitive level = **life satisfaction (domain satisfaction + bottom-up process)**	Individuals experiencing a preponderance of positive evaluations about one's life using certain standards of comparison (satisfaction with one's life compared to one's past life, the life of family members, the life of associates at work, the life of others in the same social circles, etc.) relative to negative evaluations about one's life using similar or other standards of comparison	Multiple discrepancies theory; congruity life satisfaction; temporal life satisfaction; social comparison; frequency of positive affect; homeostatically protected mood	Domain satisfaction (satisfied with work life, social life, family life, etc.) at the cognitive level mediated by a bottom-up process at the meta-cognitive level result in life satisfaction; and conversely. domain dissatisfaction (dissatisfied with work life, social life, family life, etc.) mediated by a bottom-up process result in life dissatisfaction

(continued)

Table 7.1 (continued)

Positive mental health defined at a developmental level = **eudaimonia (life satisfaction + personal growth)**	Individuals experiencing a preponderance of positive psychological traits (self-acceptance, personal growth, purpose in life, environmental mastery, autonomy, positive relations with others, etc.) relative to negative psychological traits (pessimism, hopelessness, depressive disorder, neuroticism, impulsiveness, etc.)	Hedonic versus eudaimonic happiness; virtue ethics and character strengths; self-determination theory; personal expressiveness; psychological well-being; purpose and meaning in life; flourishing; orientations to happiness; resilience; and satisfaction of the full spectrum of human needs	Life satisfaction at the meta-cognitive level mediated by a process involving high personal growth result in high levels of eudaimonia at the developmental level; and conversely, life dissatisfaction mediated by a process involving low personal growth result into low levels of eudaimonia.
Positive mental health defined at a social-ecological level = **socio-eudaimonia (eudaimonia + social & moral development)**	Individuals experiencing a preponderance of social resources (social acceptance, social actualization, social contribution, social integration, social harmony, social belonginess, social attachment, familial attachment, etc.) relative to social constraints (social alienation, social discord, social exclusion, ostracism, etc.)	Social well-being, social harmony need to belong, attachment theory; social exclusion and ostracism	High levels of eudaimonia at the developmental level mediated by a process involving high social and moral development result into high levels of socio-eudaimonia at the social-ecological level; and conversely, low levels of eudaimonia mediated by a process involving low social and moral development result into low levels of socio-eudaimonia.

10. Social growth and potential,
11. Acceptance of others,
12. Social interest and coherence,
13. Self-acceptance.

Note that the first seven dimensions of positive mental health focus on eudaimonia and other lower-order constructs of well-being. Dimensions 8-13 reflect the interface between the individual and society, and this interface must be positive to reflect positive mental health.

Allow me to elaborate on Keyes' work related to social well-being. As previously mentioned, Keyes' (1998, 2002, 2007, 2013) has articulated the most popular definition of positive mental health, namely a higher-order construct involving three dimensions: hedonic well-being, psychological well-being, and social well-being. Hedonic well-being involves positive affect, life satisfaction, as well as the absence of negative affect. This construal of hedonic well-being is essentially synonymous with subjective well-being (e.g., Diener, 1984; Diener, Suh, Lucas, & Smith, 1999). I discussed these as concepts of well-being at lower levels of analysis (emotional, cognitive, and meta-cognitive levels). As described in the preceding chapter, psychological well-being focuses on personal growth and development. It involves positive psychological traits such as personal growth, purpose in life, environmental mastery, autonomy, and positive relations with others. The construct of psychological well-being is essentially based on Ryff's (1989) model of psychological well-being. In contrast, *social well-being* reflects positive aspects of human well-being through interaction with other people and the community at large. This construct involves at least five dimensions (e.g., Keyes, 1998, 2002, 2003: Keyes & Lopez, 2002, Keyes & Waterman, 2003; Robitschek & Keyes, 2009): (1) social acceptance, (2) social actualization, (3) social contribution, (4) social coherence, and (5) social integration.

Social acceptance refers to a positive view of people and human nature. People high on social acceptance trust others, believe that generally people are kind and industrious. Socially accepting people tend to feel comfortable with others. Social acceptance is an analogue to personal acceptance, a significant dimension of eudaimonia. That is, people who accept both the good and the bad aspects of themselves.

Social actualization refers to a positive view of human society and human strivings to elevate civil society. People high on social actualization believe in the potential and the trajectory of society and humanity at large. Society and human civilization have evolved and continue to evolve in a positive way to meet the needs of humanity through institutions and responsible citizenship. Social actualizers are hopeful about the condition and future of society and recognize society's potential. They also recognize that the future generation are potential beneficiaries of societal development. Social actualization reflects the sense that we, as individuals in a given society, control our collective destiny. Social actualization is analogous to eudaimonic concepts related to self-actualization, eudaimonic happiness, and personal growth with a social twist. In other words, social actualization reflects the fundamental belief that society grows and develops to achieve its human potential.

Social contribution refers to a positive view of the need to contribute to society through good deeds. People high on social contribution believe that every human being can make some contribution to society. People are naturally productive, and everyone can give something of value to give to the world. Social contribution has its parallel in eudaimonic concepts such as efficacy and competence in a broader social context. That is, people have the ability to contribute something of value to society. Social alienation is the antonym of social contribution reflecting the perception of lack of value of one's life. Social contribution has its eudaimonic analogue to generative motives and behavior—adults are motivated by a desire to contribute to society.

Social coherence refers to a positive view of how institutions work to foster societal well-being. People high on social coherence believe in the society's norms, laws, and institutions. Social norms, laws, and institutions are established for good cause, to foster society and its functioning. People high on social coherence have a basic understanding of what is happening around them. Of course, they do not delude themselves in the belief that society and its norms, laws, and institutions is perfect. They believe that people are fallible; and so, society is equally fallible. Nevertheless, society works best when fallibility is recognized and corrected. They believe that society is discernable, sensible, and predictable to the most extent. They also see their personal lives as meaningful and coherent, a eudaimonic attribute, generalizing this fundamental belief to society also being meaningful and coherent.

Finally, *social integration* refers to a positive view of social identity and a sense of belonging to a community. It refers to one's evaluation of the quality of one's relationship to the family, community, and society at large. People high on social integration feel that they are integral to their family, the community, and society at large. They have something in common with others in their neighborhood and the greater community. Social integration is about social cohesion, the antonym of cultural estrangement and social isolation. Estrangement is the rejection of society; the realization that one doesn't belong to the group because the group does not share one's own values. Social isolation is the breakdown of personal relationships, relationships that are vital in providing moral and physical support. In sum, social integration is the belief in collective membership and the shared fate of the collective. It is about solidarity and consciousness with others.

Research has demonstrated that subjective well-being, psychological well-being, and social well-being are correlated but also empirically distinct (e.g., Gallagher, Lopez, & Preacher, 2009; Joshanloo, 2016; Joshanloo, Bobowick, & Basabe, 2016; Keyes, 2002; Keyes, Shmotkin, & Ryff, 2002; Robitschek & Keyes, 2009; Shapiro & Keyes, 2008). A measure of positive mental health/flourishing was related to several personality traits. The results indicate that positive mental health/flourishing is positively related to extraversion, conscientiousness, agreeableness, and negatively related to extraversion (Joshanloo & Nostrabadi, 2009), a pattern of findings consistent with much of the research on personality and subjective well-being (cf. Keyes, 2006a, 2006b).

Much of this discussion hints at a possible imperative, the need to take into account the social resources available in one's environment as well as social constraints. A person with optimal mental health is not only high on eudaimonia but also high on social well-being (i.e., high on social acceptance, social actualization, social contribution, social coherence, and social integration). As such, I offer a definition of positive mental health at the social-ecological level as follows: Positive mental health is a state of mind in which the individual experiences a *preponderance of social resources (social acceptance, social actualization, social contribution, social coherence, social integration, etc.) relative to social constraints (social alienation, social discord, social exclusion, ostracism, etc.).*

Social Harmony

The concept of social well-being is also consistent with a large literature in cross-cultural psychology on *social harmony* (e.g., Ho & Chan, 2009; Joshanloo & Weijers, 2014). Social harmony is important in the way the individual adapts to the environment. Social harmony can be described as social quality, which means social-economic security, social inclusion, social cohesion, and empowerment in developing the individual's potential. For example, people in collectivistic societies adapt better to their environment by engaging in behaviors considered "collective" such as teamwork and sharing credit for successful task completion and blame for task failure. Social harmony refers to a state of an individual in which he or she recognizes that behavioral control resides not only with the individual but also in contextual and social forces (Morling & Fiske, 1999). As such, the individual attempts to merge with these forces, accepting his or her role and the social norms that guide his or her performance in these roles.

Harmony is a quintessential value central among the Chinese and in Chinese culture. Chinese people view harmony as a basic goal of society. In China, the issue of social harmony has been extensively studied and debated (Li, 2010; Li, Chen, Zhang, & Li, 2008; Wang, 2007; Wang, Pan, & Lian, 2008; Wang & Tong, 2006). Biannual surveys of social harmony have been conducted in Hong Kong since 2006 by social scientists from the Chinese University of Hong Kong. The goal of this social survey has been to measure people's perceptions of social harmony in Hong Kong and the extent to which government policies are successful in establishing and maintaining social harmony. Over the years and through repeated administration, the survey results indicate that most residents in Hong Kong agree that social harmony should be the key goal of development for Hong Kong even though most perceive that Hong Kong is not harmonious at present (Ip, 2014). The survey revealed that the causes of perceived disharmony in Hong Kong include conflict between big business and citizens, conflict between government and citizens, and conflict between the rich and poor. Other less significant causes of disharmony include political conflict, familial conflict, discrimination against socially disadvantaged groups, and conflict between employees and employers. The social survey also indicated that social harmony can be achieved by

- good governance;
- good law and order and protecting individual freedoms and property;
- protection of labor rights;
- enhancing fair competition and cracking down on monopoly;
- promoting multicultural diversity;
- fostering economic development and creating jobs;
- showing compassion and care to the poor;
- strengthening family ties; and
- promoting democracy.

Ip (2014) also reported on another major social survey conducted in the city of Beijing to measure social harmony. Ip focused on select indicators to highlight the concept of social harmony, or more specifically "disharmony":

- government abusive fee charges;
- school abusive fee charges;
- land graft, unfair compensation;

- patient-doctor conflict;
- unfair court, uncivil law enforcement;
- ill-treatment of the unemployed;
- corruption, looting state assets;
- wages unpaid/withheld, long working hours;
- bad workplace, manager uncivil;
- social welfare disagreements; environmental pollution; and
- disagreements concerning big-item expenses.

As a synopsis, Ip ends up defining social harmony as a "social state which displays balance, alignment, mutual support and flourishing. It is a state that is devoid of conflicts, tensions and discords" (Ip, 2014; p. 730). A society is balanced when no single interest group becomes dominant to the extent that other interest groups become disadvantaged. Alignment is about interest groups in society working together for a common cause or purpose. Mutual support and flourishing means that members of society support each other and work together in good will and trust to help all interest groups thrive and prosper. It is a state devoid of human conflicts including conflict with nature and the environment.

Much of this discussion point to the need to consider aspects of social harmony and discord in our view of well-being and positive mental health. As such, I can define positive mental health at the social-ecological level of analysis as follows: Positive mental health is a state of mind in which the individual experiences a *preponderance of social resources (forces and conditions reflective of social harmony) relative to social constraints (forces and condition reflective of social discord).*

The Need to Belong

The concept of social well-being is also consistent with the concept of the need to belong. Specifically, Baumeister and Leary (1995) proposed the *need to belong* as a fundamental human motive that is evolutionary based and hence is prevalent across all human cultures and societies. People need to establish quality relationships with others, particularly with at least one person allowing frequent and emotionally pleasant interactions. Quality social interactions reflect an element of bonding with others—a feeling that others care about one's welfare. Quality relationships play an important role in human happiness (see Gere & MacDonald, 2010 for a review of the evidence supporting the theory of the need to belong).

Baumeister and Leary (1995) argued that because the need for belongingness is a strong in human beings, threats of social exclusion influence individuals' cognition, affective reactions, and behaviors. They hypothesized with supportive evidence that threats to belonging lead to increased cognitive focus on social connections, and too much focus on social connections may hinder effective decision making in other domains. Specifically, individuals experiencing social threats to exclusion tend to experience the following cognitive effects:

- better memory for interpersonal and social events;
- greater attention to vocal tone in speech;
- greater accuracy in reading emotions in facial expressions and other nonverbal signs of communications such as body language;
- better performance of complex cognitive tasks framed in social terms;
- worse performance on cognitive tasks not related to social relationships such as intelligence tests, recall of complex passages, and answering complex analytical questions;
- stronger beliefs in supernatural agents; and
- stronger tendency to anthropomorphize non-human agents such as animals and pets.

Evidence also suggest that individuals high on the need for belongingness tend to react to threats to social exclusion more strongly compared to individuals with less need. Specifically, they experience stronger negative emotions (e.g., anger, sadness, shame, embarrassment), lower levels of positive mood, seek reparative sources of connection, and retaliate against those parties that instigated the rejection as well as innocent bystanders.

Experiments focusing on cognitive reactions to events that suggest the possibility of future acceptance in a group have shown individuals with high need to belong tend to expend greater effort and persist more on tasks they believe may lead to group membership, experience positive affect in anticipation of their group inclusion, and seek social connections with others. In sum, when people are explicitly rejected by others, they tend to withdraw from those who have rejected them to prevent further loss of face and guarding against additional damage. However, failure in social connections can also lead to efforts to re-establish social connections. Thwarting the need for belonging repeatedly and frequently usually lead to long-term ill-being outcomes. For example, older adults who experience much rejection by others have been found to report poorer health in general, more specific health conditions, and greater functional limitations over time.

The need to belong is manifested to a great extent in marital relationships. That is, people get married because they feel the need to belong to another person, a life partner. A meta-analysis of 93 studies by Proulx, Helms, and Buehler (2007) showed that higher marital quality is associated with higher levels of well-being, concurrently and over time. Several moderating effects were also significant including gender, length of marriage, and the source of both marital quality. Specifically, the association between marital quality and well-being was stronger for wives than husbands, using concurrent measures. However, this difference between husbands and wives diminishes in longitudinal surveys. With respect to marriage duration, the meta-analysis show that marital quality is stronger for shorter than longer marriages, perhaps attributed to the honeymoon effect.

The preceding discussion suggests that social resources (such as group membership and feeling that one belongs to identity salient groups and individuals such as spouses or life partners) play a positive and important role in socio-eudaimonia. Conversely, social exclusion plays a negative role. As such, positive mental health at the social-ecological level can be construed as a state of mind in which the individual experiences a *preponderance of social resources (social inclusion and membership in identity salient groups and individuals satisfying the need for belongingness) relative to social constraints (threats of social exclusion and actual manifestation of exclusion)*.

Attachment Theory

Attachment theory (Bowlby, 1969, 1973, 1980) is another theory with its own stream of research that emphasizes the importance of social relationships, particularly parental relationships—relationship between parent and child. Personal well-being is significantly compromised in relationships characterized as low attachment with parents, particularly in children.

Attachment theory posits that the real relationships of the earliest stages of life play a very important role in shaping survival and basic human attachment lies at the center of the human experience. Schore and Schore (2008) explain why early attachment experiences impact the development of systems involved in affect and self-regulation. Specifically, attachment communication between mother and child influences structural right brain neurobiological systems involved in emotions, stress, and self-regulation. As such, resilience in the face of stress and novelty is very much a function of attachment security. Attachment relationships throughout the life span are modulated by the attachment relationship forged mother and child given the fact that early attachment experiences are fundamental to brain development and emotional regulation. Much research, according to Schore and Schore (2008), has indicated that right lateralized limbic areas of the brain are responsible, not only for the regulation of autonomic functions but also in cognitive processes related to social connections.

Mother–child attachment tend to be generalized to attachments with significant others throughout the life span. For example, a study conducted by Cicirelli (1989) showed that the well-being of older persons depends on their perception of the closeness of the sibling bond and disruption of that bond. Closeness of the bond was related to less depression. Also, perceptions of conflict in their relationships with their siblings were related to increased depression.

The research on adult attachment show that people with different attachment styles differ markedly in the quality of their love relationships (e.g., Brennan & Shaver, 1992, 1995). Adults with more of a secure style report more positive relationship experiences than those with the less-secure style. Secure adults report their relationships as intimate, stable, and satisfying. In contrast, less-secure adults report low levels of intimacy, commitment, and satisfaction. They tend to be preoccupied with issues involving jealousy, conflict, and negative emotional experiences.

Much of this discussion hints at a possible imperative, the need to consider how social resources in the form of familial support plays an important role in socio-eudaimonia. Familial support allows the individual to feel secure enough to venture out and engage the uncertain and tumultuous environment. Familial support affords the individual with emotional resources to face adversity and overcome the many obstacles in modern living. With such support the individual is paralyzed by social constraints. As such, I can define positive mental health at the social-ecological level of analysis as follows: Positive mental health is a state of mind in which the individual experiences a *preponderance of social resources (in the form of support, security, and attachment from specific familial sources such as mother, father, brother, sister, and other close family members) relative to social constraints (lack of such support from other family members).*

Social Exclusion and Ostracism

Research on *social exclusion* and *ostracism* has shown that feelings of ostracism may take a toll on happiness (Wolfer & Scheithauer, 2013). That is, well-being suffers when an individual experiences social exclusion and ostracism from salient reference groups. Human beings are biologically wired to survive and prosper in groups. Group attempts to shun, ostracize, and exclude selected members wreak havoc on the mental state of these members. In contrast, a sense of belonging to the group is an important ingredient to mental well-being. Mental well-being is enhanced when the individual experiences a sense of group acceptance and public recognition of the membership.

When ostracism persists overtime, the ostracized individuals experience alienation from the group, and they become depressed with feelings of lack of control, helplessness, and unworthiness (e.g., Lau, Moulds, & Richardson, 2009; Williams, 2001, 2009; Williams & Nida, 2016; Zadro, Williams, & Richardson, 2004). Experimental research using animals (e.g., prairie voles) show that social isolation leads to symptoms that mimic depression and learned helplessness in humans (Grippo, Wu, Hassan, & Carter, 2008). Grippo, Trahanas, Zimmerman II, Porges, and Carter (2009) found that administration of oxytocin (the social-affiliative neurochemical) can reduce the adverse effects of social isolation in prairie voles. Remember, I discussed oxytocin in the second chapter of this book in relation to the neurobiology of happiness. Oxytocin is one of the neurotransmitters associated with social bonding (cf. Cacioppo & Hawkley, 2003; Gaertner, 2009; Wesselmann, Nairne, & Williams, 2012).

Much of this discussion suggests that social exclusion in the form of ostracism takes a heavy toll of well-being. Social exclusion and ostracism can be viewed as "social constraints" as opposed to "social resources." As such, I believe that this research stream supports the following definition of positive mental health at the social-ecological level: Positive mental health is a state of mind in which the individual experiences a *preponderance of social resources (in the form of social acceptance and approval) relative to social constraints in the form of (social exclusion and ostracism).*

Emergence

Socio-eudaimonia is a well-being concept that is best understood in the context of the hierarchy of concepts of well-being, specifically at the social-ecological level of the hierarchy. Socio-eudaimonia has been the focus of this chapter. The question the reader is likely to pose is: How does eudaimonia (a developmental-level concept of well-being) contributes to the formation of socio-eudaimonia at the social-ecological level? As explained in the preceding chapters, this link can be viewed in terms of emergence. To reiterate, emergence refers to higher-level systems "emerge" from lower-level systems. In other words, complex systems have "emergent properties" that are not inherent in their individual parts and cannot be understood even with full understanding of the parts alone.

As such, socio-eudaimonia is an emergent property from the interaction between eudaimonia and a process related to social and moral development. Or more succinctly put, people high on eudaimonia are likely to place themselves in situations or environments that can produce eudaimonia in a social context characterized (i.e., "socio-eudaimonia"). To function and function well daily in the context of society at large, the individual must establish and maintain positive relations with other within the family, the community, and other people involved in society's many institutions. As such, one of the positive psychological traits of eudaimonia is positive relations with others. This trait concomitant with other eudaimonic traits serve to contribute to social well-being, a key element of socio-eudaimonia.

One popular theory of social development is that of Erik Erickson (Erikson, 1974; Erikson & Erickson, 1997; Steven, 2008). According to Erikson, the social environment plays a very important role in personal growth and identity as well as adjustment to social functioning. He theorized that people experience personal growth and adapt to the social environment in eight stages. Favorable outcomes of each stage are addressed as "virtues"—strengths considered inherent in the individual life cycle. Erikson argues successful social development is the balance of both extremes of each specific life-stage. The challenge is not to reject one polar extreme at the expense of the other. Virtue arises from the successful interplay between the two polar extremes in a life-stage. For example, "trust" and "mistrust" must both be experienced and dealt with for realistic "hope" to emerge as virtue in the first stage of social development. Similarly, "integrity" and "despair" (the two polar extreme of the last stage of development) must be embraced for "wisdom" to emerge.

The first stage (*hope: basic trust vs. basic mistrust*) covers the period of infancy (0–18 months). The infant develops basic trust or mistrust as a direct function of the quality of the maternal relationship. An important element of relationship quality at this stage is the extent to which the mother (or caretaker) provides stable and constant care. The trust that the infant develops at this stage influences social relationships other than parental. Failure to develop trust at this early stage of social development results in long-lasting fear and anxiety promulgating the sense that the world is unpredictable and therefore uncontrollable.

Stage 2 (*will: autonomy vs. shame*) covers the period of early childhood (1–3 years old). The child discovers his or her independence. Parents at this stage typically encourages the child to do things on his or her own. The child discovers his or her own skills at accomplishing basic tasks such as mastering toilet training and playing games. Conversely, discouragement undermines autonomy and self-efficacy resulting in feelings of shame and unworthiness.

Stage 3 (*purpose: initiative vs. guilt*) covers the period of preschool (3–5 years old). At this stage, children interacting with other children and engage in playful activities. They develop confidence in their ability to deal with others; hence, they develop their sense of initiative. Conversely, if their social interactions result in reprimands and punishment, they develop a sense of guilt—a sense of being a burden to others. Children at this stage are inquisitive and curious. They ask many to satisfy their need for knowledge and understanding of how the world works. Critical responses from parents and others can lead to feelings of guilt. Success in this stage translates into a sense of purpose, which is balance between initiative and guilt.

Stage 4 (*competence: industry vs, inferiority*) covers the school-age period (6–11 years old). At this stage, children develop a sense of competence by comparing their success on tasks with their peers. As such, the peer group becomes very important at this stage. They will undertake socially rewarding tasks to demonstrate their skills in various domains (academics, sports, games involving elements of mastery, etc.) Failure to demonstrate competence leads to a sense of inferiority. Competence is viewed as balance between industry and inferiority.

Stage 5 (*fidelity: identity vs. role confusion*) covers the adolescence years (12–18 years old). The focus of the stage of social development is identity formation. Adolescents at this stage question themselves to develop a sense of who they are, what they would like to become, how they fit in in the context of their social circle and the community at large. Moral beliefs are established through discovering their own personal identity. They begin to learn about the many social roles they are prepared to assume in society to successfully transition into adulthood. Adolescents at this stage try to create an identity separate and possibly different from their parents, to claim their own personhood separate from their parents. Failure to one's own persona may result into role confusion and possibly identity crisis. As such, fidelity is the ability to engage in social roles on one's own terms.

Stage 6 (*love: intimacy vs. isolation*) is essentially the first stage of adult development (18–40 years old). This stage of life is marked with dating, marriage, family, work, and friendships. Success in this stage is defined in term of successfully forming loving relationships with other people and experiencing love and intimacy. Failure at this stage results into isolation, loneliness, apathy, and perhaps personal alienation.

Stage 7 (*care: generativity vs. stagnation*) is the second stage of adulthood (40–65 years old). People are either making good progress in their careers. They are raising their children and participating in their activities. They serve their communities by becoming involved in community activities and organizations. Failure at work, family, and community leads to a sense of stagnation and social alienation.

Stage 8 (*wisdom: ego integrity vs. despair*) is the third stage of adulthood (65+ years old). People are writing the last chapters of their lives and are beginning to retire. They accept life in its fullness, what they have accomplished, the legacy they will leave behind. This is what ego-integrity is about. Failing to do so results in personal despair. They struggle with questions left unanswered, relationships riddled with conflict, and unmet life goals. This despair may lead into depression and hopelessness. Wisdom involves the feeling of living a successful life.

Why is Erickson's theory of social development important to the emergence concept? As previously mentioned, socio-eudaimonia is an emergent property from the interaction between eudaimonia and a process related to social and moral development. People high on eudaimonia successfully navigate social environments in a manner to generate socio-eudaimonia. One can assume that people high on eudaimonia have been more successful in creating virtue or balance at each of the eight stages of social development. In other words, a person high on eudaimonic well-being is likely to achieve balance between basic trust and mistrust (in the form of hope), autonomy and shame (in the form of will), initiative and guilt (in the form of purpose), industry versus inferiority (in the form of competence), identity and role confusion (in the form of fidelity), intimacy and isolation (in the form of love), generativity and stagnation (in the form of care), and ego-integrity and despair (in the form of wisdom). A person who is socio-eudaimonic is therefore characterized as a person who is high on eudaimonia and having achieved the virtues from social development (hope, will, purpose, competence, fidelity, love, care, and wisdom). That is, these virtues concomitant with other eudaimonic traits serve to contribute to social well-being, a key element of socio-eudaimonia.

Another very popular theory of social and moral development is that of Kohlberg (Kohlberg, 1958, 1971, 1973, 1976, 1981; Kohlberg, Levine, & Hewer, 1983; Levine, Kohlberg, & Hewer, 1985). The theory holds that moral development is a function of how the individual navigates the social environment and reasons in moral terms when faced with moral dilemmas. He argues that moral reasoning involves three key stages (pre-conventional, conventional, and post-conventional), and within each of these key stages there are at least two stages within.

The *pre-conventional level* of moral reasoning, common in children, involves very basic and rudimentary moral judgments based on judging the ethicality of an action based on its anticipated positive and negative consequences (i.e., personal rewards and punishment). There are two sub-stages within the pre-conventional stage, namely obedience/punishment and self-interest. In Stage 1 (*obedience/punishment*) the individual focuses on the direct consequences of their actions on themselves. An action is judged as ethical is it is rewarded by an authority figure; unethical if it leads to punishment by the authority figure. In Stage 2 (*self-interest*), the focus is on "what is in it for me." That is, an action is judged as ethical if the person stands to gain something concrete and tangible by engaging in that action. An action is judged to be unethical if it does not serve one's self-interest.

The *conventional level* of moral reasoning involves using society's norms, expectations, rules, regulations, and laws as guide to judging whether an action is deemed ethical or unethical. In other words, at this key stage of development, the individual's code of conduct is reflective or society's norms and expectations. The individual goes along with society's norms and expectations and judges his or her conduct, as well-as the conduct of others, accordingly. Two stages are embedded within the second level of moral development, namely social consensus and law and order). In Stage 3 (*social consensus*), people make judgments about a person being good or bad based on social standards and social approval and disapproval. Individuals in Stage 4 (*law and order*) believe that it is important to obey the law, customs, and other social conventions because these norms maintain the functioning of society. An action is deemed ethical if the action is in conformance with laws, custom, or social convention.

The *post conventional level* involves adherence to principles, moral dictums that are deduced by the individual through social experience. Here an individual may deem that conforming with a specific law of social convention may violate certain moral principles embraced by the individual. Hence, conformance to law and order can be deemed unethical if such behavior conflict with one's moral principles. There are two stages in the post-conventional level, namely social contract and universal ethical principles. In Stage 5 (*social contract*) the individual buys into the notion that laws, customs, and other social conventions are not absolute edicts but implicit social contracts between the individual and society. Adherence to the social contract is necessary to allow society's institutions to function; otherwise, chaos and social disorder may ensue. In Stage 6 (*universal ethical principles*), the individual develops his or her own moral code based on a studied understanding of moral philosophy and perhaps theology.

Why is Kohlberg's theory of moral development important to the emergence concept? I argue that socio-eudaimonia is an emergent property from the interaction between eudaimonia and a process related to social and moral development. The focus is on moral development in this case. When faced with moral dilemmas, people high on eudaimonia tend to be more successful in making ethical decisions in ways to further enhance social well-being, a key element in socio-eudaimonia. People high eudaimonia are likely to reach the post-conventional stage of moral development quicker than those low on eudaimonia. Moral decisions reflective of post-conventional morality serve society's interests, which in turn contribute to the individual overall sense of socio-eudaimonic well-being.

In sum, individuals high on eudaiomonia are likely to grow faster through the social and moral development stages (as described by both Erickson's and Kholberg's theories of development). Such personal growth is most likely to contribute to the transformation of the person's sense of eudaimonia to socio-eudaimonia, the ultimate and the most superordinate form of well-being. Much research has already documented the finding that eudaimonia is associated with socio-eudaimonia (e.g., Gallagher et al., 2009; Joshanloo, 2016; Joshanloo et al., 2016; Keyes, 2002; Keyes et al., 2002; Robitschek & Keyes, 2009; Shapiro & Keyes, 2008). For example, a measure of positive mental health/flourishing was related to several personality traits such as extraversion, conscientiousness, agreeableness, and negatively related to extraversion (Joshanloo & Nostrabadi, 2009; Keyes, 2006a, 2006b). The positive personality traits can be viewed as eudaimonic traits reflective of personal growth and development. Based on the preceding discussion, one can argue that *high levels of eudaimonia at the developmental level mediated by a process involving high social and moral development result*

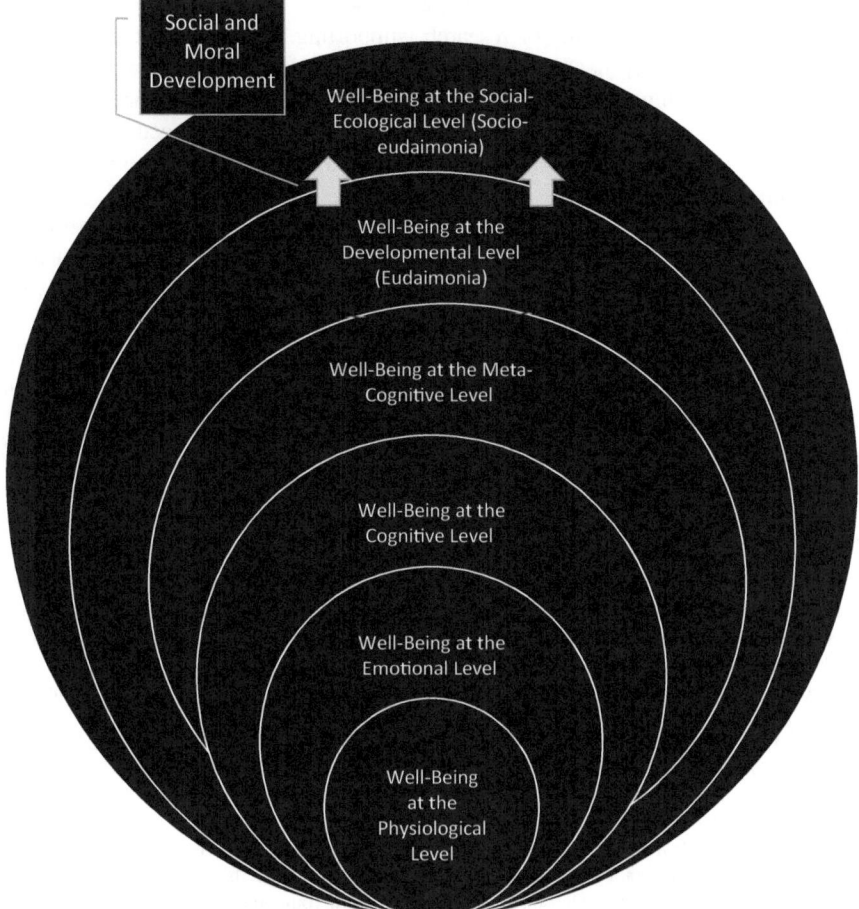

Fig. 7.1 Emergence: well-being at the social-ecological level (socio-eudaimonia) influenced by well-being at the developmental level (eudaimonia) mediated by a process of social and moral development

into high levels of socio-eudaimonia at the social-ecological level; and conversely, low levels of eudaimonia mediated by a process involving low social and moral development result into low levels of socio-eudaimonia. See Figure 7.1.

Conclusion

A definition of positive mental health based on the concept of positive balance at the social-ecological developmental was presented in this chapter. Individuals characterized as high in positive mental health tend to experience a preponderance of social resources (social acceptance, social actualization, social contribution, social integration, etc.) relative to social constraints (social exclusion, ostracism, etc.). I then discussed five programs of research, supporting this definition: social well-being, social harmony need to belong, attachment theory; social exclusion and ostracism. Following this discussion, I described how positive balance expressed in socio-eudaimonia (at the social-ecological level) is produced in part by eudaimonia (at the developmental level) mediated by a process involving social and moral development.

The next chapter will offer some concluding thoughts. I'll provide the reader a brief synopsis of the theory. I will then discuss the emerging trend in positive psychology, coined as the "Second Wave" followed by a discussion of well-accepted definitions of quality of life, health, and mental well-being. In doing so I'll compare the definitions to the definitions introduced in this book. Lastly, I'll compare selected models of mental health that involve hierarchical concepts of quality of life to my proposed theory.

References

Bauer, J. J. (2016). Eudaimonic growth: The development of the goods in personhood (or: Cultivating a good life story). In J. Vitterso (Ed.), *Handbook of eudaimonic well-being* (pp. 147–174). Dordrecht: Springer.

Baumeister, R. F., & Leary, M. R. (1995). The need to belong: Desire for interpersonal attachments as a fundamental human motivation. *Psychological Bulletin, 117*, 497–523.

Bowlby, J. (1969). Disruption of affectional bonds and its effects on behavior. *Canada's Mental Health Supplement, 59*, 12.

Bowlby, J. (1973). *Attachment and loss (Separation, anxiety, and anger)* (Vol. 2). New York: Basic Books.

Bowlby, J. (1980). *Attachment and loss (Loss)* (Vol. 3). New York: Basic Books.

Brennan, K. A., & Shaver, P. R. (1992). Attachment styles and the "big five" personality traits: Their connections with each other and with romantic outcomes. *Personality and Social Psychology Bulletin, 18*, 536–545.

Brennan, K. A., & Shaver, P. R. (1995). Dimensions of adult attachment, affect regulation, and romantic relationship functioning. *Personality and Social Psychology Bulletin, 21*, 267–283.

Cacioppo, J. T., & Hawkley, L. C. (2003). Social isolation and health, with an emphasis on underlying mechanisms. *Perspectives in Biology and Medicine, 46*, S39–S52.

Carlquist, E., Ulleberg, P., Delle Fave, A., Nafstad, H. E., & Blakar, R. M. (2017). Everyday understandings of happiness, good life, and satisfaction: Three different facets of well-being. *Applied Research in Quality of Life, 12*, 481–505.

Cicirelli, V. G. (1989). Feelings of attachment to siblings and well-being in later life. *Psychology and Aging, 4*, 211–216.

Diener, E. (1984). Subjective well-being. *Psychological Bulletin, 95*, 542–575.

Diener, E., Suh, E. M., Lucas, R. E., & Smith, H. L. (1999). Subjective well-being: Three decades of progress. *Psychological Bulletin, 125*, 276–302.

Erikson, E. H. (1974). *Dimensions of a new identity*. New York: W. W. Norton & Company.

Erikson, E. H., & Erickson, J. M. (1997). *The life cycle completed* (extended ed.). New York: W. W. Norton & Company.

Gaertner, L. A. (2009, October). *A bio-social model of positive ingroup regard: Oxytocin as an evolved hormonal mediator of intragroup social-regulation*. Presented at the Society for Experimental Social Psychology, Portland, ME.

Gallagher, M. W., Lopez, S. J., & Preacher, K. J. (2009). The hierarchical structure of well-being. *Journal of Personality, 77*, 1025–1049.

Gere, J., & MacDonald, G. (2010). An update of the empirical case for the need to belong. *The Journal of Individual Psychology, 66*, 93–115.

Grippo, A. J., Trahanas, D. M., Zimmerman II, R. R., Porges, S. W., & Carter, C. S. (2009). Oxytocin protects against negative behavioral and autonomic consequences of long-term social isolation. *Psychoneuroendocrinology, 34*, 1542–1553.

Grippo, A. J., Wu, K. D., Hassan, I., & Carter, C. S. (2008). Social isolation in prairie voles induces behaviors relevant to negative affect: Toward the development of a rodent model focused on co-occurring depression and anxiety. *Depression and Anxiety, 25*, E17–E26.

Ho, S. S. M., & Chan, R. S. Y. (2009). Social harmony in Hong Kong: Level, determinants, and policy implications. *Social Indicators Research, 91*, 37–58.

Ip, P.-K. (2014). Harmong as happiness? Social harmony in two Chinese societies. *Social Indicators Research, 117*, 719–741.

Joshanloo, M. (2016). Revisiting the empirical distinction between hedonic and eudaimonic aspects of well-being using exploratory structural equation modeling. *Journal of Happiness Studies, 17*, 2023–2036.

Joshanloo, M., Bobowick, M., & Basabe, N. (2016). Factor structure of mental well-being: Contributions of exploratory structural equation modeling. *Personality and Individual Differences, 102*, 107–110.

Joshanloo, M., & Nostrabadi, N. (2009). Levels of mental health continuum and mental health traits. *Social Indicators Research, 90*, 211–224.

Joshanloo, M., & Weijers, D. (2014). Aversion to happiness across cultures: A review of where and why people are averse to happiness. *Journal of Happiness Studies, 15*, 717–735.

Keyes, C. L. M. (1998). Social well-being. *Social Psychology Quarterly, 61*, 121–140.

Keyes, C. L. M. (2002). The mental health continuum: From languishing to flourishing in life. *Journal of Health and Social Behavior, 43*, 207–222.

Keyes, C. L. M. (2003). Complete mental health: An agenda for the 21st century. In C. L. M. Keyes & J. Haidt (Eds.), *Flourishing: Positive psychology and the life well-lived* (pp. 293–312). Washington, DC: American Psychological Association.

Keyes, C. L. M. (2006a). Subjective well-being in mental health and human development research worldwide: An introduction. *Social Indicators Research, 77*, 1–10.

Keyes, C. L. M. (2006b). Mental health in adolescence: Is America's youth flourishing? *The American Journal of Orthopsychiatry, 76*, 395–402.

Keyes, C. L. M. (2007). Promoting and protecting mental health as flourishing: A complementary strategy for improving national mental health. *American Psychologist, 62*, 95–108.

Keyes, C. L. M. (Ed.). (2013). *Mental well-being: International contributions to the study of positive mental health*. Dordrecht: Springer.

Keyes, C. L. M., & Lopez, S. J. (2002). Toward a science of mental health: Positive directions in diagnosis and interventions. In C. R. Snyder & S. J. Lopez (Eds.), *The handbook of positive psychology* (pp. 45–59). New York: Oxford University Press.

Keyes, C. L., Shmotkin, D., & Ryff, C. D. (2002). Optimizing well-being: The empirical encounter of two traditions. *Journal of Personality and Social Psychology, 82*, 1007–1022.

Keyes, C. L. M., & Waterman, M. B. (2003). Dimensions of well-being and mental health in adulthood. In M. Bornstein, L. Davidson, C. L. M. Keyes, & K. A. Moore (Eds.), *Well-being: Positive development throughout the life course* (pp. 481–501). Mahwah, NJ: Erlbaum.

Kohlberg, L. (1958). *The development of modes of thinking and choices in years 10 to 16*. Ph.D Dissertation, University of Chicago.

Kohlberg, L. (1971). *From is to ought: How to commit the naturalistic fallacy and get away with it in the study of moral development*. New York: Academic.

Kohlberg, L. (1973). The claim to moral adequacy of a highest stage of moral judgment. *Journal of Philosophy, 70*, 630–646.

Kohlberg, L. (1976). Moral stages and moralization: The cognitive-developmental approach. In T. Lickona (Ed.), *Moral development and behavior: Theory, research and social issues*. Holt, NY: Rinehart and Winston.

Kohlberg, L. (1981). *Essays on moral development* (The philosophy or moral development) (p. 1). San Francisco, CA: Harper & Row.

Kohlberg, L., Levine, C., & Hewer. (1983). *Moral stages: A current formulation and response to critics*. Base, NY: Karger.

Lane, R. E. (1991). *The market experience*. Cambridge: Cambridge University Press.

Lane, R. E. (1994). Quality of life and quality of persons: A new role for government? *Political Theory, 22*, 219–252.

Lane, R. E. (1996). Quality of life and quality of persons: A new role for government? In A. Offer (Ed.), *The pursuit of the quality of life* (pp. 256–294). New York: Oxford University Press.

Lane, R. E. (2000). *The loss of happiness in market democracies*. New Haven, CT: Yale University Press.

Lau, G., Moulds, M. L., & Richardson, R. (2009). Ostracism: How much it hurts depends on how you remember it. *Emotion, 9*, 430–434.

Levine, C., Kohlberg, L., & Hewer, A. (1985). The current formulation of Kohlberg's theory and a response to critics. *Human Development, 28*, 94–100.

Li, P. L. (Ed.). (2010). *Livelihood of contemporary China*. Beijing: Social Sciences Documentation Publication. (in Chinese).

Li, P. L., Chen, K. J., Zhang, Y., & Li, W. (2008). *China's social harmony and stability report*. Beijing: Social Sciences Documentation Publication. (in Chinese).

Morling, B., & Fiske, S. T. (1999). Defining and measuring harmony control. *Journal of Research in Personality, 33*, 379–414.

Proulx, C. M., Helms, H. M., & Buehler, C. (2007). Marital quality and personal well-being: A meta-analysis. *Journal of Marriage and Family, 69*, 576–593.

Robitschek, C., & Keyes, C. L. M. (2009). Keyes's model of mental health with personal growth initiative as a parsimonious predictor. *Journal of Counseling Psychology, 56*, 321–329.

Ryff, C. D. (1989). Happiness is everything, or is it? Explorations on the meaning of psychological well-being. *Journal of Personality and Social Psychology, 57*, 1069–1081.

Schore, J. R., & Schore, A. N. (2008). Modern attachment theory: The central role of affect regulation in development and treatment. *Clinical Social Work Journal, 36*, 9–20.

Shapiro, A., & Keyes, C. L. M. (2008). Marital status and social well-being: Are the married always better off? *Social Indicators Research, 88*, 329–346.

Steven, R. (2008). *Erik Erickson: Explorer of identity and the life cycle*. Basingstoke, England: Palgrave Macmillan.

Wang, C. K. (2007). *The basic problems of the theory of socialist harmonious society*. Beijing: People's Publication. (in Chinese).

Wang, C. K., Pan, W., & Lian, S. (2008). *Thirty years of values change in Chinese society*. Beijing: Social Sciences Publication. (in Chinese).

Wang, Y. H., & Tong, S. J. (2006). *Harmonious society from a multi-disciplinary perspective*. Shanghai: Xue Lin Publication. (in Chinese).

Wesselmann, E. D., Nairne, J. S., & Williams, K. D. (2012). An evolutionary social psychological approach to studying the effects of ostracism. *Journal of Social, Evolutionary, and Cultural Psychology, 6*, 309–328.

Williams, K. D. (2001). *Ostracism: The power of silence*. New York: The Guilford Press.

Williams, K. D. (2009). Ostracism: Effects of being excluded and ignored. In M. Zanna (Ed.), *Advances in experimental social psychology* (pp. 275–314). New York: Academic.

Williams, K. D., & Nida, S. A. (Eds.). (2016). *Ostracism, exclusion, and rejection*. New York: Taylor & Francis.

Wolfer, R., & Scheithauer, H. (2013). Ostracism in childhood and adolescence: Emotional, cognitive, and behavioral effects of social exclusion. *Social Influence, 8*, 1–20.

Zadro, L., Williams, K. D., & Richardson, R. (2004). How low can you go? Ostracism by a computer is sufficient to lower self-reported levels of belonging, control, self-esteem, and meaningful existence. *Journal of Experimental Social Psychology, 40*, 560–567.

Chapter 8
Concluding Thoughts

Introduction

> Well-being cannot exist just in your own head. Well-being is a combination of feeling good as well as actually having meaning, good relationships and accomplishments.—Martin Seligman (https://www.brainyquote.com/topics/well-being-quotes)

As a reminder and a reinforcer, a brief synopsis of the theory will be provided to the reader. Following the synopsis, I discuss the emerging trend "Second Wave in Positive Psychology," after which I discuss two well-accepted definitions of quality of life, health, and mental well-being. I then compare these definitions to my definition of positive mental health at the various hierarchical levels. Finally, I compare selected models of mental health that involve hierarchical concepts of quality of life to my own model to highlight the contribution of my model in the extant literature.

A Synopsis of the Theory

The theory of positive balance of well-being and positive mental health can be summarized as follows.

At the *physiological* level, well-being is construed in terms of positive and negative neurochemicals. The positive neurochemicals are associated with the brain reward center, whereas negative neurotransmitters are associated with the stress response system. Positive balance is defined at the physiological level as follows: Individuals with high levels of positive mental health are characterized to experience a preponderance of neurochemicals related to positive emotions (dopamine, serotonin, etc.) relative to neurochemicals related to negative emotions (cortisol). This definition of positive mental health at the physiological level is supported

© Springer Nature Switzerland AG 2020
M. J. Sirgy, *Positive Balance*, Social Indicators Research Series 80,
https://doi.org/10.1007/978-3-030-40289-1_8

by much research related to the stress response system and the neurobiology of happiness (see Table 8.1).

At the *emotional* level, well-being is viewed in terms of positive and negative affect. Positive balance is defined as follows: Individuals with high levels of positive mental health are characterized to experience a preponderance of positive affect (happiness, joy, etc.) relative to negative affect (anger, sadness, etc.). This definition is supported by much research related to the distinction between positive versus negative affect, the broaden and build theory of positive emotions, and flow theory (see Table 8.1).

At the *cognitive* level, well-being is treated as domain satisfaction. Positive balance is defined as follows: Individuals with high levels of positive mental health are characterized to experience a preponderance of domain satisfaction (satisfaction in salient and multiple life domains such as family life, work life, etc.) relative to dissatisfaction in other life domains. This definition is supported by much research related to three major principles, namely satisfaction limits, the full spectrum of human developmental needs, and diminishing satisfaction (see Table 8.1).

At the *meta-cognitive* level, well-being is conceptualized as life satisfaction. Positive balance is defined as follows: Individuals with high levels of positive mental health are characterized to experience a preponderance of a preponderance of domain satisfaction (satisfaction in salient and multiple life domains such as family life, work life, etc.) relative to dissatisfaction in other life domains. This definition is supported by much research related to multiple discrepancies theory, congruity life satisfaction, temporal life satisfaction, social comparison, and frequency of positive affect (see Table 8.1).

At the *developmental* level, well-being is construed as eudaimonia. Positive balance is defined as follows: Individuals with high levels of positive mental health are characterized to experience a preponderance of positive psychological traits (self-acceptance, personal growth, etc.) relative to negative psychological traits (pessimism, hopelessness, etc.). This definition is supported by much research related to the distinction between hedonic and eudaimonic happiness, virtue ethics and character strengths, self-determination theory, personal expressiveness, psychological well-being, purpose and meaning in life, flourishing, orientations to happiness, and satisfaction of the full spectrum of human need (see Table 8.1).

At the *social-ecological* level, well-being is construed as socio-eudaimonia. Positive balance is defined as follows: Individuals with high levels of positive mental health are characterized to experience a preponderance of perceived social resources (social acceptance, social actualization, etc.) relative to perceived social constraints (social exclusion, ostracism, etc.). This definition is supported by much research related to social well-being, social harmony need to belong, attachment theory, and social exclusion and ostracism (see Table 8.1).

Furthermore, I have argued that well-being at each hierarchical level contributes to a higher-order construct of well-being from the physiological level all the way up to the social-ecological level. Specifically, well-being at the physiological level (positive and negative neurotransmitters) plays a key role in the formation of well-being at the emotional level (positive and negative affect). That is, positive

Table 8.1 Positive mental health defined at various hierarchical levels as positive balance with emergence

Level of analysis	Positive balance as positive mental health	Programs of research	Emergence
Positive mental health defined at a physiological level = **positive and negative neurotransmitters**	Individuals experiencing a preponderance of neurochemicals related to positive emotions (dopamine, serotonin, oxytocin) relative to neurochemicals related to negative emotions (cortisol)	Stress response system); neurobiology of happiness)	
Positive mental health defined at an emotional level = **positive/ negative affect or hedonic well-being (positive/negative neurotransmitters + cognitive appraisals)**	Individuals experiencing a preponderance of positive emotions (happiness, joy, serenity, contentment, etc.) relative to negative emotions (anger, sadness, jealousy, envy, depression, etc.)	Positive versus negative affect; broaden and build theory; flow	Positive neurochemicals (dopamine, serotonin, and oxytocin) at the physiological level mediated by a process of cognitive appraisal (positive frame) result into positive affect (happiness, joy, contentment, etc.) at the emotional level; and conversely, negative neurochemicals (cortisol) mediated by a process of cognitive appraisal (negative frame) result into negative affect (anger, sadness, jealousy, envy, depression, etc.)
Positive mental health defined at a cognitive level = **domain satisfaction (positive/negative affect + domain segmentation)**	Individuals experiencing a preponderance of domain satisfaction (satisfaction in salient and multiple life domains such as family life, work life, social life, etc.) relative to	Principle of satisfaction limits; principle of the full spectrum of human developmental needs; principle of diminishing satisfaction	Positive affect (happiness, joy, contentment, etc.) at the emotional level mediated by a process of domain segmentation result into domain satisfaction (satisfied with

(continued)

Table 8.1 (continued)

Level of analysis	Positive balance as positive mental health	Programs of research	Emergence
	dissatisfaction in other life domains		work life, social life, family life, etc.); and conversely, negative affect (anger, sadness, jealousy, envy, depression, etc.) mediated by a process of domain segmentation result into domain dissatisfaction (dissatisfied with work life, social life, family life, etc.)
Positive mental health defined at a meta-cognitive level = **life satisfaction (domain satisfaction + bottom-up process)**	Individuals experiencing a preponderance of positive evaluations about one's life using certain standards of comparison (satisfaction with one's life compared to one's past life, the life of family members, the life of associates at work, the life of others in the same social circles, etc.) relative to negative evaluations about one's life using similar or other standards of comparison	Multiple discrepancies theory; congruity life satisfaction; temporal life satisfaction; social comparison; frequency of positive affect; homeostatically protected mood	Domain satisfaction (satisfied with work life, social life, family life, etc.) at the cognitive level mediated by a bottom-up process at the meta-cognitive level result in life satisfaction; and conversely. Domain dissatisfaction (dissatisfied with work life, social life, family life, etc.) mediated by a bottom-up process result in life dissatisfaction
Positive mental health defined at a developmental level = **eudaimonia (life satisfaction + personal growth)**	Individuals experiencing a preponderance of positive psychological traits (self-acceptance, personal growth, purpose in life, environmental mastery,	Hedonic versus eudaimonic happiness; virtue ethics and character strengths; self-determination theory; personal expressiveness; psychological well-being;	Life satisfaction at the meta-cognitive level mediated by a process involving high personal growth result in high levels of eudaimonia at the developmental

(continued)

Table 8.1 (continued)

Level of analysis	Positive balance as positive mental health	Programs of research	Emergence
	autonomy, positive relations with others, etc.) relative to negative psychological traits (pessimism, hopelessness, depressive disorder, neuroticism, impulsiveness, etc.)	purpose and meaning in life; flourishing; orientations to happiness; resilience; and satisfaction of the full spectrum of human needs	level; and conversely, life dissatisfaction mediated by a process involving low personal growth result into low levels of eudaimonia.
Positive mental health defined at a social-ecological level = **socio-eudaimonia** **(eudaimonia + social & moral development)**	Individuals experiencing a preponderance of social resources (social acceptance, social actualization, social contribution, social integration, social harmony, social belongingness, social attachment, familial attachment, etc.) relative to social constraints (social alienation, social discord, social exclusion, ostracism, etc.)	Social well-being; social harmony; need to belong; attachment theory; social exclusion and ostracism	High levels of eudaimonia at the developmental level mediated by a process involving high social and moral development result into high levels of socio-eudaimonia at the social-ecological level; and conversely, low levels of eudaimonia mediated by a process involving low social and moral development result into low levels of socio-eudaimonia.

neurochemicals (dopamine, serotonin, and oxytocin) at the physiological level mediated by a process of cognitive appraisal result into positive affect (happiness, joy, contentment, etc.) at the emotional level; and conversely, negative neurochemicals (cortisol) mediated by a process of cognitive appraisal result into negative affect (anger, sadness, jealousy, envy, depression, etc.). Moving up one notch in the well-being hierarchy, the theory posits that well-being at the emotional level (positive and negative affect) plays a key role in the formation of well-being at the cognitive level (domain satisfaction). That is, positive affect (happiness, joy, contentment, etc.) at the emotional level mediated by a process of domain segmentation results into domain satisfaction (satisfied with work life, social life, family life, etc.); and conversely, negative affect (anger, sadness, jealousy, envy, depression, etc.)

mediated by a process of domain segmentation results into domain dissatisfaction (dissatisfied with work life, social life, family life, etc.). Another notch up the hierarchy is well-being at cognitive level (domain satisfaction). The theory states that domain satisfaction plays a key role in the formation of well-being at the meta-cognitive level (life satisfaction). That is, domain satisfaction (satisfied with work life, social life, family life, etc.) at the cognitive level mediated by a bottom-up process at the meta-cognitive level results in life satisfaction; and conversely, domain dissatisfaction (dissatisfied with work life, social life, family life, etc.) mediated by a bottom-up process results in life dissatisfaction. Moving on up to well-being at the developmental level (eudaimonia), the theory states that well-being at the meta-cognitive level (life satisfaction) plays an important part in the formation of eudaimonia. That is, life satisfaction at the meta-cognitive level mediated by a process involving high personal growth results in high levels of eudaimonia at the developmental level; and conversely, life dissatisfaction mediated by a process involving low personal growth results into low levels of eudaimonia. Focusing on the most superordinate concept of well-being, the proposition is that well-being at the developmental level (eudaimonia) plays a major role in the formation of socio-eudaimonia. That is, high levels of eudaimonia at the developmental level mediated by a process involving high social and moral development result into high levels of socio-eudaimonia at the social-ecological level; and conversely, low levels of eudaimonia mediated by a process involving low social and moral development result into low levels of socio-eudaimonia.

The reader is likely to further appreciate the proposed theory by knowing something about the trend in positive psychology research, referred to as the "Second Wave." We will now turn to this discussion.

Second Wave Positive Psychology

The concept of *positive balance* is consistent with much of the discussion of "Second Wave Positive Psychology" (Lomas, Hefferon, & Ivtzan, 2015; Lomas & Ivtzan, 2016). Second Wave Positive Psychology is an emerging movement within positive psychology that acknowledges the problems inherent in treating positive mental health concepts as either "positive" or "negative." As such, the movement recognizes the dialectical nature of positive mental health—a complex and dynamic interplay of positive and negative mental states. As succinctly captured by Ryff and Singer (2003, p. 272), well-being involves "inevitable dialectics between positive and negative aspects of living."

The concept of positive mental health as extracted from the positive psychology movement has been criticized because of its overemphasis on individualism and positive thinking. For example, Ehrenreich (2009) has asserted that positive psychologists preaching the concept of positive mental health, based on individualism and positive thinking and set apart from the larger culture, have overpromised the public. They overpromised to transform people's lives by merely thinking positively while ignoring what should be changed in the environment to help change people's lives. The social environment plays a significant role in the make-up of well-being. Of course, if we strictly focus on the individual without understanding how the environment affects positive mental health then there should be no call to action on the political front. The positive psychology movement implies that life coaches and therapists advise their clients and patients to change themselves by changing their thought pattern. Instead, to enhance positive mental health much can be done to change social institutions. Other critics have voiced similar concerns (e.g., Allen, 2018; Davies, 2016; Held, 2002, 2005). The concept of well-being introduced here takes into account many disciplinary aspects of the discourse on mental well-being—aspects from physiology, the study of emotions, cognitive science, human development, and sociology. I hope that my conceptualization of mental well-being can guide future research and public policy.

I will now discuss well-established definition of quality of life, health, and mental well-being vis-à-vis the concepts of positive balance as proposed throughout this book. My hope is that this comparative analysis will further elevate readers' appreciation of the proposed theory.

Definitions of Quality of Life, Health, and Mental Well-being

One can compare our definition of positive mental health with two popular definitions, namely the World Health Organization's definition of quality of life (WHO, 1997) and Galderisi, Heinz, Kastrup, Beezhold, and Sartorius (2015) definition published in *World Psychiatry*. The World Health Organization (WHO) defines quality of life as:

> Individuals' perception of their position in life in the context of the culture and value systems in which they live and in relation to their goals, expectations, standards and concerns. It is a broad ranging concept affected in a complex way by the person's physical health, psychological state, level of independence, social relationships, personal beliefs and their relationship to salient features of their environment (WHO, 1997, p. 1).

My definition of positive mental health is consistent with WHO's definition of quality of life in that it takes into account aspects from physiology ("physical health" as mentioned in WHO's definition), psychology ("individuals; perception," "goals, expectations, standards and concerns," and "psychological state" in WHO's definition), and sociology ("level of independence, social relationships, personal beliefs and their relationship to salient features of their environment" as mentioned in WHO's definition). These are consistent with my definition which covers the entire hierarchical gamut: quality of life aspects viewed from different levels of analysis: physiological, emotional, cognitive, meta-cognitive, developmental, and social-ecological. My definition of positive mental health is better than WHO's definition because the concepts I use stem from a long tradition of research on health-related quality of life and well-being. As such, the definition of positive mental health offered in this book serves to integrate much of the literature in a systematic way.

Galderisi et al. (2015) developed a definition of positive mental health which is also consistent with my integrative and hierarchical definition.

> Mental health is a dynamic equilibrium which enables individuals to use their abilities in harmony with universal values of society. Basic cognitive and social skills; ability to recognize, express and modulate one's own emotions, as well as empathize with others; flexibility and ability to cope with adverse life events and function in social roles; and harmonious relationship between body and mind represent important components of mental health which contribute, to varying degrees, to the state of internal equilibrium (pp. 231–232).

The definition emphasizes "internal equilibrium," the individual's use of abilities "in harmony with universal values of society," and "harmonious relationship between body and mind." My definition also emphasizes "balance," "equilibrium," homeostasis," and a preponderance of certain positive over negative aspects identified at different levels of analyses (physiological, emotional, cognitive, meta-cognitive, developmental, and social-ecological). Hence, my definition is more integrative in the sense that it covers a large gamut of concepts of positive mental health discussed at various hierarchical levels. In contrast to Galderisi et al.'s definition of mental health, my definition of positive mental health emphasizes the notion of *positive balance*. That is, positive mental health is not simply a balanced state, static or dynamic; it involves a preponderance of certain desired states above and beyond undesirable states, reflective of the "positive" nature of the balanced state. As such, I believe that my definition of positive mental health is not only integrative but also provides a different perspective on mental health. *It builds on the concept of balance but also acknowledges the positivity of the balanced state.*

I will now discuss models involving hierarchical concepts of quality of life. Doing so, may further enhance readers' appreciation of the proposed theory.

A Comparison of Models Involving Hierarchical Concepts of Quality of Life

My hierarchical model of positive mental health can be compared to other models promulgating a hierarchical approach to quality-of-life concepts. These models include Wilson and Cleary (1995), Dambrun et al. (2012), Huta and Waterman (2014), and Lomas et al. (2015).

The Wilson/Cleary Model

Wilson and Cleary (1995) fleshed out relationships among measures of patient outcomes in a health-related quality-of-life conceptual model. The quality-of-life construct is, in essence, is on top of the hierarchy. At the bottom of the hierarchy is the construct capturing *biological and physiological variables* associated with, perhaps, a disease such pulmonary tuberculosis as detected and confirmed by pulmonary function tests. This disease is manifested in terms of *symptom status* (the patient's physical and psychophysical symptoms associated with pulmonary tuberculosis). These physical and psychophysical symptoms are likely to interfere with daily functioning (the ability of the individual to perform particular tasks on a daily basis). This is referred to as *functional status.* Hindrance in daily functioning plays a direct and important role in the individual's *general perception of health,* which, in turn, strongly influences the individual's quality of life (e.g., life satisfaction). The model is designed to help medical personnel and health-related quality-of-life researchers connect patient-related outcomes, and it certainly does a good job with that task. However, the model does not deal directly with positive mental health and the hierarchy of quality-of-life concepts involving positive mental health, concepts such as stress, allostasis, neurochemicals related to positive emotions (dopamine, serotonin, etc.) and negative emotions (cortisol), the psychology of positive and negative emotions, life satisfaction, domain satisfaction, psychological well-being (or eudaimonia), and social well-being.

The Dambrun Model

Dambrun et al. (2012) also used a hierarchical dimension varying from "fluctuating happiness" to "authentic-durable happiness" to make a clear distinction between hedonic well-being and eudaimonic well-being. *Fluctuating happiness* is viewed as a micro-level concept that is ephemeral, temporary, and transient, whereas *authentic-durable happiness* is regarded as dispositional, stable, and enduring across a larger time frame. As such, they developed measures capturing fluctuating happiness versus authentic-durable happiness. They were able to establish the reliability of these measures (high internal consistency and satisfactory test-retest) and validity too (adequate convergent and discriminant validity and relationships with various related constructs such as biological markers of stress). This distinction between fluctuating happiness and authentic-durable happiness is highly consistent with the hierarchical model of positive mental health. My model treats constructs related to fluctuating happiness (e.g., positive and negative affect, domain satisfaction) as lower-level constructs that fluctuate as a function of the situation, compared to constructs related to authentic-durable happiness (e.g., psychological well-being, social well-being). The latter constructs are stable and "durable." Furthermore, my model goes way beyond these two constructs to incorporate other constructs at various levels of analysis.

The Huta/Waterman Model

Huta and Waterman (2014) made a clear distinction between eudaimonia (personal growth, purpose in life, character and virtue, etc.) and hedonia (positive and negative emotions, absence of distress, etc.) based on a continuum in which the polar extremes are "state-like concepts" (most micro) to "trait-like concepts" (most macro). They argue that constructs related to hedonic well-being tend to be state-like whereas constructs reflective of eudaimonic well-being are trait-like. This distinction between hedonia and eudaimonia is highly consistent with my hierarchical model. My model treats constructs related to hedonia (e.g., positive and negative affect, domain satisfaction, and life satisfaction) as lower-level constructs that are much state-like, compared to constructs related to eudaimonia (e.g., psychological well-being, social well-being). The latter constructs are viewed to be similar to stable dispositions or personality traits. As observed in relation to the Dambrun model, my model goes way beyond these two constructs to incorporate other constructs at various levels of analysis.

The Lomas/Hefferon/Ivtzan Model

Lomas et al. (2015) proposed a model of Positive Psychology Interventions (PPI) using a layering scheme they call the LIFE model. The model involves three key dimensions (subjective/mind, objective/body, and social), with each dimension containing five layers. The layers involved with the subjective/mind dimension are embodied sensations (most micro), followed by emotions, cognitions, conscious awareness (most macro). The layers involved with the objective/body dimension are biochemistry (most micro), followed by neurons, neural networks, nervous system, and the body at large (most macro). The social dimension also involves five hierarchical layers: microsystem (most micro), followed by mesosystem, exosystem, macrosystem, and ecosystem (most macro). The goal of the LIFE model is to identify and classify the positive psychology interventions (PPIs). For example, there are PPIs targeting emotions (e.g., emotion management skills) or cognitions (e.g., gratitude journal). These can be classified as such in terms of the subjective/mind dimension. PPIs related to body-mind therapy (breathing and stress reduction techniques) can be classified as "embodied sensations." Using the objective/body dimension of the LIFE model, PPIs can be classified similarly. For example, a treatment such as serotonin reuptake inhibitor is a PPI classified as a "biochemistry" PPI. Neurofeedback is another example of PPI classified at the "neural network" level. Turning to the social dimension, PPIs focused on the individual can be classified as "mesosystem" interventions. Interventions that involve a group of collective (e.g., family's shared values) could be classified at higher hierarchical levels, perhaps at the "exosystem" level.

The LIFE model is indeed a good taxonomy that allows PPI researchers to classify specific interventions. In doing so, they may be able to identify gaps in system levels to help them develop more PPIs to fill those gaps. However, the model does not do what my positive mental health model does, namely identify the various quality-of-life/well-being constructs directly related to positive mental health. My constructs are organized hierarchically, showing the connections between each hierarchical layer explicitly. The goal here is to define positive mental health in explicit terms at each level of the hierarchy: physiological, emotional, cognitive, meta-cognitive, developmental, and social-ecological.

Conclusion

As discussed in this chapter, I believe that the concept of *positive balance* is consistent with much of the discourse of "Second Wave of Positive Psychology." The movement recognizes the dialectical nature of positive mental health—a complex and dynamic interplay of positive and negative mental states. The concept of positive mental health as promulgated in this book is in sync with the Second Wave. The Second Wave acknowledges that the social environment plays a significant role in the make-up of well-being; hence it rejects the total focus being on the individual, positive thinking, and positive emotions. It is important to account for the effects of the social environment to issue a call to action, politically speaking. The concept of well-being introduced here integrates many disciplinary aspects of the discourse on mental well-being—aspects from physiology, the study of emotions, cognitive science, human development, and sociology. I hope that my conceptualization of positive mental health can guide future research and be embraced as a call to action for public policy.

References

Allen, J. (2018). *The psychology of happiness in the modern world*. New York: Springer.

Dambrun, M., Ricard, M., Despres, G., Drelon, E., Gibelin, E., Gilbelin, M., et al. (2012). Measuring happiness: From fluctuating happiness to authentic-durable happiness. *Frontiers in Psychology, 3*, article 16.

Davies, W. (2016). *The happiness industry: How the government and big business sold us well-being*. London, UK: Verso.

Ehrenreich, B. (2009). *Bright-sided: How the relentless promotion of positive thinking has undermined America*. New York: Metropolitan Books.

Galderisi, S., Heinz, A., Kastrup, M., Beezhold, J., & Sartorius, N. (2015). Toward a new definition of mental health. *World Psychiatry, 14*, 231–233.

Held, B. S. (2002). The tyranny of the positive attitude in America: Observation and speculation. *Journal of Clinical Psychology, 58*, 965–992.

Held, B. S. (2005). The "virtues" of positive psychology. *Journal of Theoretical and Philosophical Psychology, 25*, 1–34.

Huta, V., & Waterman, A. S. (2014). Eudaimonia and its distinction from hedonia: Developing a classification and terminology for understanding conceptual and operational definitions. *Journal of Happiness Studies, 15*, 1425–1456.

Lomas, T., Hefferon, K., & Ivtzan, I. (2015). The LIFE model: A meta-theoretical conceptual map for applied positive psychology. *Journal of Happiness Studies, 16*, 1347–1364.

Lomas, T., & Ivtzan, I. (2016). Second wave positive psychology: Exploring the positive-negative dialectics of wellbeing. *Journal of Happiness Studies, 17*, 1753–1768.

Ryff, C. D., & Singer, B. (2003). Ironies of the human condition: Well-being and health on the way to mortality. In L. G. Aspinwall & U. M. Staudinger (Eds.), *A psychology of human strengths* (pp. 271–287). Washington, DC: American Psychological Association.

Wilson, I. B., & Cleary, P. D. (1995). Linking clinical variables with health-related quality of life: A conceptual model of patient outcomes. *The Journal of the American Medical Association, 273*, 59–65.

World Health Organization. (1997). *WHOQOL: Measuring quality of life.* Geneva, Switzerland: World Health Organization, Programme on Mental Health, Division of Mental Health and Prevention of Substance Abuse.